9-4-19

SEXY
IN 6

SEXY IN 6

SCULPT YOUR BODY WITH THE
6 MINUTE QUICK-BLAST WORKOUT

TRACEY MALLETT

Da Capo Lifelong

A Member of the Perseus Books Group

New York

Text copyright © 2008 by Tracey Mallett
Photography copyright © 2008 by Dorit Theis
Photo on page 1 © Scott Ashton Photography

DESIGN BY JANE RAESE
Set in 12-point Bulmer

Cataloging-in-Publication data for this book is available from the Library of Congress.

First Da Capo Press edition 2008
ISBN-13: 978-1-60094-030-9
ISBN-10: 1-60094-030-7

Published by Da Capo Press
A Member of the Perseus Books Group
www.dacapopress.com

Note: The information in this book is true and complete to the best of our knowledge. This book is intended only as an informative guide for those wishing to know more about health issues. In no way is this book intended to replace, countermand, or conflict with the advice given to you by your own physician. The ultimate decision concerning care should be made between you and your doctor. We strongly recommend you follow his or her advice. Information in this book is general and is offered with no guarantees on the part of the authors of Da Capo Press. The authors and publisher disclaim all liability in connection with the use of this book.

Da Capo Press books are available at special discounts for bulk purchases in the United States by corporations, institutions, and other organizations. For more information, please contact the Special Markets Department at the Perseus Books Group, 2300 Chestnut Street, Suite 200, Philadelphia, PA 19103, or call (800) 255-1514, or e-mail special.markets@perseusbooks.com.

10 9 8 7 6 5 4 3 2 1

To Chris, Amber & Ty who make my life complete

CONTENTS

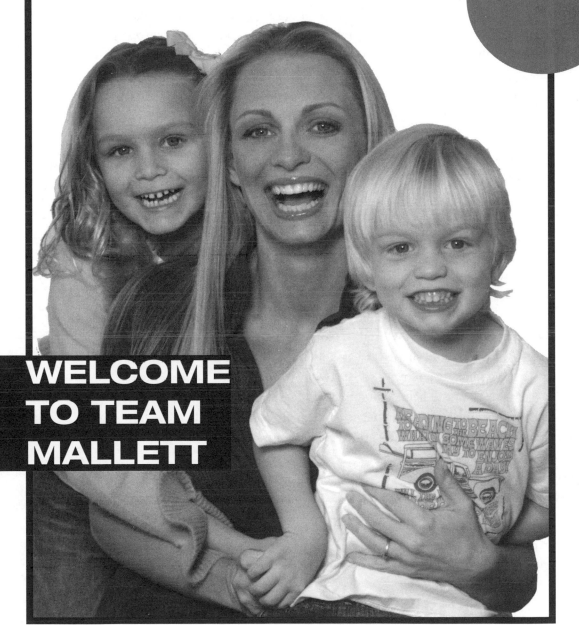

WELCOME
TO TEAM
MALLETT

"TODAY IS THE FIRST DAY OF THE REST OF YOUR LIFE." I'VE ALWAYS liked that saying because it means you can start fresh, right here and right now. In the world of fitness and weight loss, it means last week's missed gym days don't matter and yesterday's pint of Ben & Jerry's that you downed in one sitting is forgotten. You have a clean slate. Because you've picked up this book, you want to make some changes. And you can, no matter where you are in your life or what your level of fitness. You *can* change things for the better. And I'm here to help.

Feeling fit, strong, and healthy affects everything in your life—way beyond getting into your favorite bathing suit. (Although who doesn't love that?) When you feel good about your body, your relationships with your family and friends are better. Your career is better. Why? You like yourself!

TRACEY'S STORY

I've been a fitness trainer for nearly twenty years—I started doing this when I was in college. That was back in the eighties, when wearing leg warmers and striped leotards to the gym was cool. (What *were* we thinking?) Although I tossed my bright-colored Lycra leggings years ago, my desire to help people shape up has only intensified. It's something I'm seriously passionate about.

Why do I want to help so much? Well, I've been one of those women on the other side of the body image fence. A woman who didn't love herself. A woman who constantly criticized what she saw in the mirror. I had

MOTIVATION FROM TEAM MALLETT

I love that I can break my exercise time down into bite-sized chunks and still know it's effective. It's such a relief to know that I don't have to find an entire hour to exercise. With three kids and work, I have to utilize the time I have. I did my abs before breakfast, did my conditioning after lunch, and walked while my kids were at Kung Fu in the afternoon. In the past, I wouldn't have believed that a little bit of exercise was enough. But now that 11 pounds have melted away, I'm more than convinced!
— Sally Teiniker, 32, Auckland, New Zealand

been a dancer my entire life, and being a performer means all eyes are on you. I was striving to be perfect, always comparing myself to the bodies and lives of famous women and finding that mine didn't add up. But over time, I've worked hard to love and accept who I am. And I've made lots of realizations along the way.

I started dancing as a toddler and have always been active. But it was in my teen years that I realized the importance of health. It was back then that my mother's youngest sister, Susan, died of breast cancer. She was just 33 years old and had a 2-year-old daughter. As you can imagine, this was devastating—but it got worse. Within the next year, my mother and another of her sisters were both diagnosed with breast cancer. Four years later, a fourth sister found out she had the disease. I felt like a walking time bomb. Fitness was not part of my family's lifestyle, but the more I learned about its link to good health, the more important it became to me. I knew that I couldn't do anything about my genes, but I could focus on the things that were in my control: diet and exercise.

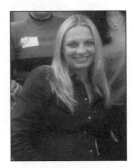

Can you believe this is me with 50-plus pounds on my little frame?

I was on a mission for wellness. So when I took my first conditioning class and was introduced to Pilates and body sculpting, I was hooked. I loved how fun the exercises were and how they improved my dance performance. I also loved my toned, lean muscles. But most of all, I loved how strong and confident the exercises made me feel—proud of my body instead of critical. I wanted to show other women how they could feel that way, too. That's when I started teaching and training clients. Nothing was as exciting as getting people off the couch, away from the fridge, and into their sweats. I still feel that way today when I watch as clients change their bodies and, thus, their lives.

When I was thirty, just after the birth of my first child, researchers in England who were studying my family history identified the specific breast cancer gene that ran in my family. It was a big moment, but a scary one, too. I was shaking in my shoes, but I headed to the City of Hope Hospital in Los Angeles to take the test that would determine whether I'd face the same fate as my mother and my aunties. Now *I* was a mother and I felt that I owed it to my daughter—and myself—to find out.

I waited six long weeks for the test results. I'll never forget the day I got the good news that I did not carry the breast cancer gene. I can honestly say that the world became a different place for me. It made me even more determined to help myself and other women stay as healthy as possible and be more appreciative of what they have: Life!

I am telling you all this so you know why I wanted to write this book. I have helped women through the thousands of DVDs I've sold worldwide and my programs on *Exercise TV,* a popular on-demand channel. I do the same with my personal training clients at my studio in Los Angeles. But through a book, I can explain my philosophy and give more hands-on, detailed help than I can on a DVD. But lucky you! You get the best of both worlds because I've enclosed a DVD with the book.

THE SEXY IN 6 PLAN

Before writing this book, I got together a group of ninety women and put them through the plan you'll find in these pages. The women ranged from ages 26 to 60, with different body types and different goals. Some were aiming for a big weight loss, others were trying to lose those last 10 pounds, and some were just looking to get more toned. The two things they had in common was that they were short on time and weren't big on exercise. These ladies, who I call Team Mallett, were an inspiring and amazing group. Together, they lost almost 400 pounds!

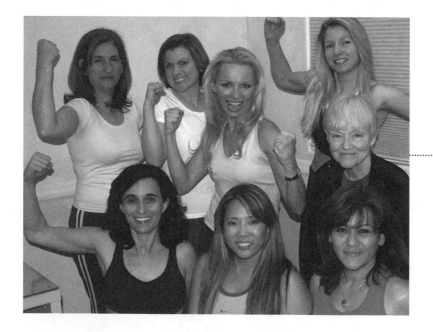

But their transformations were more than skinny-jeans deep. I saw their confidence level rise. I saw how their relationships with their husbands, children, and friends changed. More importantly, I saw how their love and respect for themselves changed. They felt happy and confident. They felt sexy. They wanted to get dressed up and go out and feel good. They weren't going to hide in the corner and be wallflowers. Each one found a woman inside who she didn't even know existed. Okay, my corny side is coming out, but I can tell you that I was in tears more than once while reading their weekly progress reports. Look for their results and success stories throughout the book; they're *beyond* inspiring. (I had room to highlight only fourteen of these women, who lost a total of 179 pounds and 144.5 inches!)

I'm a working mom whose life consists of juggling two young kids, my clients, my business, contributions to various women's magazines, and, oh yeah, my husband. I developed the *Sexy in 6* plan over years of working with real women just like you, women who have busy lives and are multitasking from the second they get up until their heads hit the pillow at night. My fitness plan doesn't try to change your schedule; it's made to fit right into it.

The *Sexy in 6* workouts are all six-minute morsels. I am not saying that you can lose weight and get the body you want in six minutes a day. That's a gimmick and I don't believe in those. What I *am* saying is that by squeezing these segments in throughout the day, you can get in shape. With *Sexy in 6*, you can choose one or more six-minute segments and do them in the morning, afternoon, night—whenever you have time. On days when you're short on time, do less; on days when you suddenly have an hour to yourself, do a lot more. The big myth is that you need one hour a day to exercise or it's not worth it. Wrong! You can make a positive effect on your body in small, bite-sized chunks of time throughout the day.

For a more detailed description of the plan, see chapter 3, "The Sexy in 6 Exercise Plan." For specific workout combinations that target different areas of your body, see chapter 2, "Working Out for Your Body Type."

The keys to making a change are consistency and effective, efficient exercises. I'm living proof of that and so are all my clients and the lovely ladies who make up Team Mallett. In fact, many of them said that the most surprising part of my program was that small spurts of exercise throughout the day really do reap great results.

IT'S ABOUT HEALTH, NOT PERFECTION

Most of us are searching for an unrealistic body and are too influenced by the perfect body images we see in the media. Oftentimes, what we're looking for is unachievable due to the high standards we place on ourselves. We have the gift of being able to create the miracle of life, yet we stop living ours in fear of accepting ourselves. We think, *why bother, it's too hard*. But one key thing I've learned is that beauty and health have nothing to do with a dress size and everything to do with how you feel on the inside. Now, being in good shape on the outside helps that by elevating your confidence. I like to think of the body as a work in progress, and the goal is not perfection but a healthy body and mind.

MOTIVATION FROM TEAM MALLETT

What I really like about this program is the consistency. There's a little something to do each morning and it's all planned out for me. All I have to do is wake up and put on my clothes! I am so grateful that after just four weeks I got my waist back and my arms have much less jiggle!
—Diane Kelber Guillory, 52, Los Angeles, California

GET READY TO GET RESULTS!

All this brings me back to how I can help you. After all, you picked up this book to help yourself, not hear my life story. But there's one more thing I'd like to share.

Although I had always been fit and trim thanks to dancing, I was in for a shock after my first child was born. I packed 55 pounds on my 5-foot 3-inch frame during that pregnancy. I wasn't worried *while* I was pregnant because I was in shape. Of course that weight—almost half my original body size—would magically melt away after my daughter was born thanks to breastfeeding, right? Oh, so wrong! I struggled to shed those pounds just like the rest of you moms. It was downright depressing to realize that someone whose day job is fitness didn't have a slim-down-fast pass to post-pregnancy. I worked my butt off—literally—and it was tough. However, the experience helped me refine my fitness philosophy and made me realize even more how important it is to live a healthy life, not starve oneself or hop on the latest diet or fitness bandwagon. I had to come up with a plan—a plan for life.

Now that I've chatted your ear off, it's time to reveal the plan that I promise is going to fit seamlessly into your life and take you where you want to go, physically and mentally. Just think of me as your best girl-friend with a bunch of fitness degrees under her belt. So lace up those sneakers, get ready, and follow me.

Tracey's Tips

The only person responsible for your body is you. That's a big lesson I've learned over the years. *You* have to take responsibility. *You* have to be your biggest fan and cheerleader. *You* have to keep reinforcing that you can do it. Repeat to yourself, "I'm hot. I'm on the path to success. I'm sexy." You'll feel silly at first, but who cares? This is between you and, well, just you. When you start seeing changes in your body, you'll believe every word of it!

Success Story

∙∙

My mom, Lynne Jones, 54, Pasadena, California

Lost

16 lbs

6 percent body fat

One dress size

5 inches off her waist

6 inches off her hips

2 inches off her thighs

13 inches total

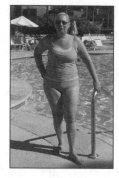 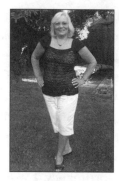

Before   After

Gained

Respect for her body. *My body has been through so much with all the surgeries and medications I've had to take because I had breast cancer. Instead of giving up on it like I did in the past, it feels so good to be taking care of and appreciating my body.*

● ● ● ● ●

Although my mom, Lynne Jones, joined the program to support me (something she's done my whole life. Thanks mom!), she also needed to lose some weight. She said she had been a yo-yo dieter since the day I was born! "I ballooned to 185 pounds during my pregnancy and over the next twenty years my weight fluctuated up and down depending on whether I wanted to lose weight for a special occasion," she says. "A wedding or holiday was always my motivation. After it was over, my weight went back up." Although she'd go for the occasional swim, Mom also didn't like to exercise.

When Mom had her breast cancer scare fifteen years ago, she had a mastectomy, and any desire to trim down vanished. "After undergoing major surgery, I thought that was it," she says. "Why did I need to lose weight and be attractive? My body was scarred for life and would never be the same again, so why bother?" When she had her breast reconstruction surgery, she felt better about herself, but went back to her yo-yo dieting ways to trim down. Two years ago, through gene testing, she found out that she had a fifty percent chance of getting ovarian cancer. Her doctor advised her to have her ovaries removed. "My body went back into menopause—something I'd already been through once with the chemo and drugs I'd taken," she says.

When she moved from England to the United States seven months ago, Mom's friends joked that once she moved to L.A. she'd become part of the fitness scene here. I didn't expect her to start toting a yoga mat or hire a personal trainer, but I *was* hoping her new surroundings would inspire her to live a healthier life. Extra pounds increase your risk of an array of diseases, and she's been through more than her share of those. Luckily, I was recruiting women for Team Mallett just as she was starting to think about shedding pounds for good.

Just because I was leading the program didn't mean she got an easier version of it. Like I've said before, there's no get-fit-fast pass for any of us. "The main issue for me was working out," Mom said. "Exercise was a real dirty word to me and one that I had avoided for many, many years with many, many excuses!" But once she started, Mom was stunned that she actually liked moving her body and breaking a sweat. Now regular exercise is part of her life. It's amazing and thrilling to both of us, but even more thrilling is that this time she is doing this for her. "For the first time, my goal isn't to fit into a dress for a wedding or to look good for the holidays," she says. "My goal is to look and feel good for *me!* Tracey's program gave me the will to want to succeed."

Mom's eating habits also needed a makeover. In England, she was a huge fan of Indian dishes that were high in fat. She's given that up and now eats more fresh fruit as well as low-fat snacks such as sugar-free Jell-O. All her hard work has paid off—Mom feels better than ever and is seeing results. "Now when I sit in the car, I have room on either side of my thighs because my butt and legs aren't spreading out and covering the whole seat," she says. In addition to all the pounds she's lost, she shed

LYNNE'S STICK-WITH-IT TIP

Start now. Look after your body and it will look after you.
Give your body the tools to live a long, healthy life. It's never too late!

inches from her waist and thighs. "I'm also starting to feel my abs— something I haven't been able to do since Tracey was born thirty-five years ago! When I first saw them, I couldn't believe I had muscles under all the excess weight I'd been carrying around," she says. "I need to lose another 10 to 15 pounds, but gone are my days of yo-yo dieting. Now I know that if I follow the plan, I *will* reach my goal. Most of all, being fit and toned makes me see my body as something strong and healthy, not something scarred and damaged." And that, as they say, is priceless!

TRACEY'S TAKE

I'm very proud of Mom because I know that exercising was a huge challenge for her but she powered through it with determination. For years, I've been trying to encourage her (okay, push her) to be consistent with exercise because I knew that was the key to helping get her metabolism back on track. It's been frustrating, but I now realize that she was the one who needed to make that decision, not me.

My secret plan was to get her hooked on exercise when she moved to the States. The plan worked and she's now regularly breaking a sweat with her buddy. Mom used to be a stress eater, but now she's learned to mellow her mind with exercise, not food. I'll always be here to make sure she keeps it up. I was her biggest fan before she started the program. Now I'm cheering even louder!

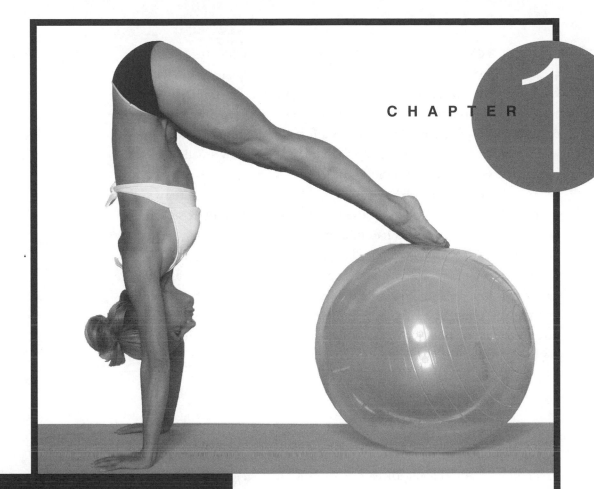

CHAPTER 1

GETTING STARTED

L ET'S GET THIS PARTY STARTED. I KNOW WHAT YOU'RE THINKING. "Party? What party?" But this *is* a party because it's a celebration of the new healthy life you're about to embark on. If that's not a reason to whoop it up, I don't know what is. Before I launch into the specific workout plans, you need to do a few things to get ready. Don't worry; they're simple—just a little shopping to buy a few small pieces of equipment (such as free weights and a ball).

You also need to record your weight and measurements. I know this isn't exciting—in fact, many of the women on Team Mallett said they were cursing me when they had to face all those numbers. But the good news is, you'll love me in six weeks. (They *swore* they did.) Why? Because those numbers will be concrete evidence of all the progress you've made: the pounds lost, the inches that have melted away. So think of this as a starting point and imagine a slimmer, leaner you in six weeks. Who cares how big the number is? It's between you and you. No one else. Being honest will only make your great results that much sweeter. Now, let's talk about what you're going to need.

FREE WEIGHTS

I recommend purchasing three sets of dumbbell weights—3, 5, and 8 pounds—because some areas of the body are strong and require heavy weights, while others are weaker and require lighter ones. Being able to vary the weight keeps all your muscles challenged and less prone to injury. Also, having different weights on hand is helpful as you get stronger and can lift more. If expense is an issue, choose between the 3 pound and the 5 pound. Note that when finishing your repetitions is too easy, it's time to use heavier weights for that exercise.

FIT BALL

A fit ball is my favorite tool for conditioning the body, especially for working on your core and balance. Fit balls come in different sizes: 55 cm is recommended for women 5 feet 5 inches and under, and 65 cm for women over 5 feet 5 inches. The ball needs to be pumped up until it's firm. To do this, you can either buy a pump or use the pump at your local gas station. Check out Appendix C for online stores that sell fit balls.

TERRIFIC TUNES

Music is a big motivator. Sometimes, great new tunes in my iPod have helped my workout go by super fast. Other times, when I have had nothing to listen to, my workout seemed to drag on. When doing strength workouts, you can simply put on some great CDs. For cardio, such as running or walking, you may want to invest in an iPod or MP3 player. Also, it's important to note that your body will naturally go to the beat of the music. So save the sultry love songs for the bedroom and use upbeat music for your cardio workout. You'll be surprised at how much harder you work to good upbeat tunes. They will inspire you!

HOW TO MEASURE CORRECTLY

Chest: Place the tape measure around your breasts and in line with your nipples.

Waist: Measure around your waist in line with your belly button.

Hips: Measure below the boney part of your hip bones (approximately 3 to 4 inches from your waist). In other words, measure the widest part of your hips, including your butt.

Arms: Measure around the middle of your upper arm between your shoulder and the elbow. Don't forget to measure both arms.

Thighs: Measure around the widest part of each thigh.

MOTIVATION FROM TEAM MALLETT

The biggest thing that got me through the program was telling people what I was doing and asking them to hold me accountable. That way, if I slipped up, I had a support team to encourage me. But most of all, I knew that if I blew it big time or quit I would have to tell everyone and disappoint them as well as myself. It really worked! Even my 7-year-old daughter was a source of support. When I first started the plan, she'd ask me why I was exercising every night. A few weeks into it, she'd ask what kind of exercise I would be doing next. Last week, when I was taking a night off, she said, "Shouldn't you be exercising?"
—*Tanya Torforson, 28, Bruderheim, Canada*

Use Music to Keep Your Cardio Workouts Fresh

Following is a sample of how you can put together songs that will help motivate you during a cardio workout. As I always say in class, "The music is your road."

INTENSITY	MUSIC TEMPO	YOUR PACE	MUSIC DURATION	MPH
Warm-up	Mid-tempo	Comfortable, light pace	1 song, 3–4 minutes	5.0
Running	Up-tempo	Increase pace by 10%	1 song, 3–4 minutes	6.0–6.5
Jog	Mid-tempo	Decrease pace until you feel comfortable	2–3 songs, 6–12 minutes	5.0–5.5
Running	Up-tempo	Increase pace by 10%	1 song, 3–4 minutes	6.0–7.0
Cool down, light jog	Mid-tempo	Decrease pace gradually	2 songs, 6–7 minutes	5.0
Walk	Mid-tempo	Continue to decrease pace	1 song, 2 minutes	3.0

Tracey's Favorite Cardio Tunes

1. *Promiscuous* by Nelly Furtado
2. *Fable* (message version) by Robert Miles
3. *Waiting for Tonight* by Jennifer Lopez
4. *Super Massive Black Hole* by Muse
5. *Independent Women* by Destiny's Child
6. *Get This Party Started* by Pink
7. *I'm Just a Girl* by Gwen Stefani
8. *Ain't No Other Man* by Christina Aguilera
9. *Never Again* by Kelly Clarkson
10. *Crazy in Love* by Beyonce
11. *Vertigo* by U2
12. *Livin' la Vida Loca* by Ricky Martin
13. *Slide* by Goo Goo Dolls

Tracey's Favorite Retro Cardio Music

(This is where I show my age.)

1. *Let's Groove Tonight* by Earth Wind & Fire
2. *The Reflex* by Duran Duran
3. *Material Girl* by Madonna
4. *Everybody Wants to Rule the World* by Tears for Fears
5. *I Feel Love* by Donna Summer

6. *It's Raining Men* by The Weather Girls
7. *Girls Just Want to Have Fun* by Cyndi Lauper
8. *Let's Hear It for the Boy* by Deniece Williams
9. *Heaven Is a Place on Earth* by Belinda Carlisle
10. *Jump (for My Love)* by The Pointer Sisters
11. *All Night Long* by Lionel Richie
12. *My Prerogative* by Bobby Brown

Tracey's Favorite Strength-Training Tunes
(These are slower paced.)

1. *Hollaback Girl* by Gwen Stefani
2. *Hips Don't Lie* by Shakira
3. *Waiting on the World to Change* by John Mayer
4. *Smooth* by Santana
5. *Ain't Nobody* by Chaka Khan
6. *Bend & Break* by Keane
7. *Photograph* by Def Leppard
8. *SOS* by Rihanna
9. *It Ain't Over 'Til It's Over* by Lenny Kravitz
10. *Things That Make You Go Hmmm* by C+C Music Factory
11. *Kiss* by Prince
12. *A New Day Has Come* by Celine Dion

Tracey's Tips

1. Download or burn your favorite songs to match the duration of your workout.

2. Vary the beats of the songs. For example, song one is for your warm-up, so choose a mid-tempo song.

3. Our bodies naturally gravitate to the beat of the music, so keep that in mind when selecting the music.

MOTIVATION FROM TEAM MALLETT

The last two weeks, I was traveling to London, China, and Tokyo for work. My hotels didn't had gyms and the rooms were tiny. But I brought my yoga mat, exercises, and DVDs with me. I even used water bottles as weights. I did the Quick-Blast DVD this morning using my laptop. When it came time for the Quick Mind-Body Blast, I had to angle my legs into the bathroom doorway to avoid hitting the wall for the dolphin kicks! I'm not sure whether the guests in the floor below me appreciated my early morning workout, but I felt great afterwards! It's proof that you really can fit in this workout anytime, anywhere.
—*Laurie Jardin, 43, Ontario, Canada*

RATE OF PERCEIVED EXERTION

Gauging how your body feels is important in evaluating how much effort you're putting into your workout. There are many methods for measuring this, but I like the Rate of Perceived Exertion (RPE) chart and the talk test together. I find that this is the easiest approach to listening to your body during your workouts.

The talk test is a subjective scale and an effective tool if you're just starting an exercise plan or have a pulmonary condition such as asthma. During aerobic exercise, you should be able to breathe comfortably, regardless of the intensity. A good way of imagining how you should feel is "comfortably uncomfortable." I know that sounds weird, but it's true. A sign of overexertion is the inability to count or string words together to form sentences. For advanced exercisers, you will be hitting RPE level 8 during anaerobic intervals. You'll be able to talk but probably no more than 10–15 words in a thirty-second interval.

This is a good way to monitor your exertion in the cardio segments of your exercise. Here's what the numbers will tell you as you're working out. Listen to your body and, with practice, you will be able to safely monitor your exertion.

RPE 1–2: Very easy; you can talk without any effort.
RPE 3: Easy, you can talk with almost no effort.
RPE 4: Moderately easy, you can talk comfortably without effort.
RPE 5: Moderate, requires some effort to talk.
RPE 6: Moderately hard, requires a bit more effort to talk.
RPE 7: Difficult, requires a lot of effort to talk.
RPE 8: Very difficult, requires maximum effort to talk.
RPE 9–10: Maximum effort, no talking.

SAFE SOLES

Although most of the *Sexy in 6* workouts can be done with little to no equipment, you must invest in a good pair of sneakers. Here are some tips from Kraig Kobayashi, the manager of team training and walking footwear at Asics America Corporation.

1. Strength training mostly involves building up muscles to increase their capacity. Therefore, choose shoes that help keep your feet stable so that energy is not wasted trying to keep your balance. Look for firmer, wider, and lower-profile midsoles.

2. For activities that involve heel strikes, such as running or walking, look for some type of heel-cushioning component that absorbs shock, such as gel.

3. The most important thing that many people overlook in their sneakers is fit. A good fit means you should never have to think about your shoes while working out. Try on a variety of models and brands. Different models, even within the same brand, have different fit characteristics.

TEN WAYS TO BOOST YOUR MOTIVATION

1. Have a plan at all times. Try to schedule your workouts the day before or, better yet, the whole week. I know this is hard when you have a busy life, but without at least a loose plan you will find it difficult to be consistent, which can lead to failure.

2. Don't procrastinate. Think about that Nike saying, "Just do it!" The earlier in the day that you work out, the more time you have throughout the day to focus on your family, work, or yourself without constantly thinking, "I need to exercise." We've all been there, putting off

TIPS FROM THE PROS

Lisa Delaney, author of *Secrets of a Former Fat Girl,* lost a whopping 70 pounds and has kept it off for twenty years. Here are two of my favorite tips from her book.

Think: "It's not an option." As In, "It's not an option to quit my workout or to have another slice of pizza." Simple as it sounds, this little mantra helped me shut off a whole world of possibility, a world where giving up and pigging out were not just acceptable, but the norm.

Don't do nothing. Doing something physical is better than doing nothing at all. Can't squeeze in thirty minutes on the treadmill? Take the fifteen minutes you do have. Lunchtime walk rained out? Then climb the stairs in your office building for twenty minutes.

exercising until finally we're too tired and can't be bothered. I could kick myself for wasting so much time procrastinating! If you just do it, it's over before you know it!

3. Focus on that fabulous post-sweat-session feeling. Think of how good you're going to feel *after* your workout and how much energy it will give you for the rest of the day. Remember you always finish a workout feeling better than you did when you started (and you can't say that about many things in life). Repeat that to yourself when your motivation lags or energy wanes.

4. Good things come in small packages. There may be days when you can fit in only one six-minute segment's worth of exercise. Go for it! Don't blow it off because you think it's not worth it. Everything adds up. It's like tossing a small handful of change into a jar every night. In a few weeks and months, those little bits of money add up. The same is true for little bits of exercise. Every calorie burned and every fiber stimulated is getting you one step closer to your goal and the hot body that *will* be yours. Think of the big picture! Tiny steps will get you there.

5. Be patient. I know how impatient you can be with yourself when you're trying to slim down. You want it to happen as soon as possible and feel bummed out when it doesn't. But from my experience, I know that the more you stay focused on the overall goal of total weight loss, the easier it is to accept that your abs aren't turning fab as quickly as you'd like. Stick with the *Sexy in 6* plan and the weight *will* come off.

6. Look on the bright side. Celebrate your positive efforts and don't get frustrated. When you feel like you're not getting anywhere, take a look at an old photo or an old pair of pants that you were wearing at your heaviest. It's empowering to see how much weight and how many inches you have lost.

7. Be realistic. Remember that muscle weighs more than fat. Judge by how your clothes fit and not by the numbers on the scale. We all have an unrealistic weight in our head—probably set from our late teens to early twenties—that we want to hold onto. Let it go and be realistic. Limit weighing yourself to once a week—even if you feel that you've lost weight. There's something about scales that can turn your plan south and leave you with little confidence.

8. Stay optimistic. I know sometimes this can be hard, but how you feel and react to circumstances has a big effect on your outcome. Instead of saying, "I'll try" say, "I will do it." Early on, I knew which Team Mallett members would be success stories just from their optimistic approach. They were true believers. Now it's your turn!

9. Count your blessings. Focus on what you do have, not what you don't. Think of problems as setbacks, not as failures. If you overeat at your sister's wedding, don't dwell on it or beat yourself up. Instead, find a solution such as dancing to burn it off!

10. Have a support system. On your own, it's too easy to get distracted when the going gets tough. Everyone needs a team of people to gently guide them through the highs and lows. It will also make you feel accountable to someone besides yourself. Tell your family, coworkers, and close friends that you're on the *Sexy in 6* program. You may even find someone to do it with you. The more people who are out there rooting for you, the more you will not want to disappoint them. Go tell the world!

TUNE YOUR MIND-BODY CONNECTION

Now it's time to ask yourself a few questions—some hard, some not so hard. As long as you're honest, there are no right or wrong answers. No one is going to see what you write except you, and if you can't be honest with yourself, then who can you be honest with? This is about you—not your kids or your husband, but you. Remember her? The person who is usually at the bottom of the list because she's busy taking care of everyone else? Sound familiar? I thought so!

Your answers make a great baseline for the *Sexy in 6* plan and a nice way to reflect and to measure your progress throughout the program. First answer the questions, and then put them away for six weeks. At the end of the program, answer them again and then compare the two. Trust me, if you're honest with yourself, you'll be so proud of how far you've come weeks from now. Take a few minutes to truthfully answer the following questions.

1. How many days a week and for how long do you exercise?
2. Do you feel like you currently eat healthy? What is your biggest food vice that you see as an obstacle?

3. What is the first thing that goes through your head when you look in the mirror?
4. Do you like what you see when you look in the mirror?
5. How do you feel when you have to get dressed up for a social event?
6. Do you generally feel sexy?
7. Do you have a strong sex drive?
8. How much energy do you have (on a scale of 1–10, with 10 the highest energy level and 1 little or no energy)?
9. Do you experience dips of energy throughout the day? If so, at what time?
10. What is your biggest reason for not exercising?
11. Do you think you can find eighteen minutes a day to exercise and follow a healthy diet plan?
12. Have you had previous successes at losing weight? If so, what was the main reason you gained the weight back?
13. If you could change one of your bad habits, what would it be?
14. What kind of changes do you hope to see in yourself in six weeks doing this plan?
15. What are your long-term health and fitness goals?
16. Are you motivated and committed to making healthy changes to your lifestyle?

PROGRESS CHART

Photocopy the progress chart (found in Appendix A) three times or download it from www.traceymallett.com. Be sure to fill it out every other week; I recommend doing so at the same time and on the same day of the week for consistency. Midweek is usually the best day because on weekends we tend to splurge. If you can't wait two weeks to weigh yourself, there's no harm doing it once a week—but *no more* than once. Often the number on the scale doesn't reflect your true progress (perhaps you're carrying water, or you ate too much salt, or the time of the month is to blame) and you can get discouraged.

ANATOMY 101

1. Traps (upper back)
2. Lats (sides of the upper back)
3. Deltoids (shoulders)
4. Rhomboids (middle of the upper back)
5. Biceps (front of the upper arms)
6. Triceps (back of the upper arms)
7. Pectorals (chest)
8. Abdominals (belly)
9. Obliques (sides of waist)
10. Quads (front of upper legs)
11. Hamstrings (back of upper legs)
12. Glutes (butt)
13. Calves (back of lower legs)

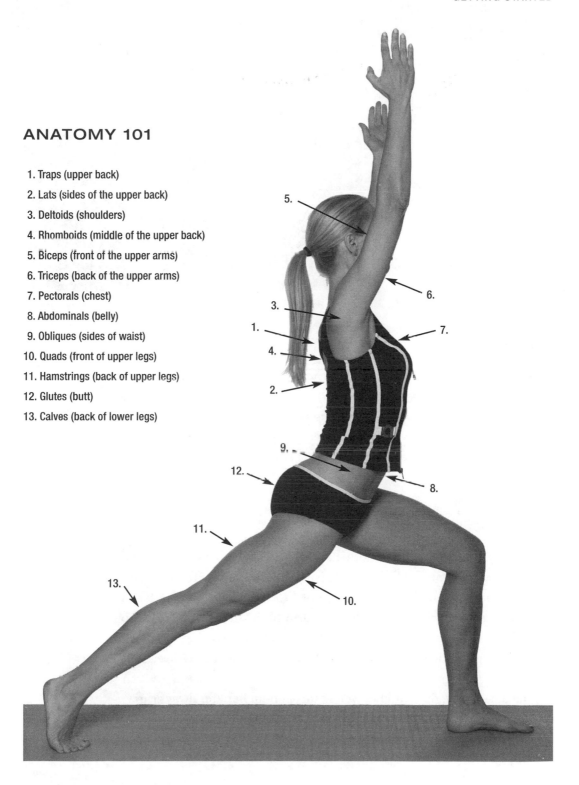

Success Story

Dana Davy-Bench, 27, Elk Grove, California

Lost

88 pounds with Tracey's DVDs

9 pounds on this program

Six dress sizes

3 inches off her arms

2½ inches off her waist

1½ inches off her hips

4 inches off her legs

11 inches total

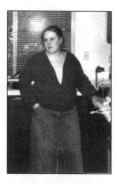
Before

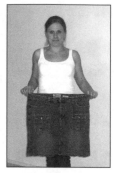
After

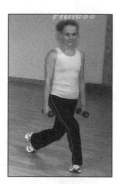
Final

Gained

A new lease on life. *When I was heavy, I was insecure and hated going anywhere. I rarely left the house or even put on makeup. Now I love going places and knowing that people look at me and think, "She looks great!" I'm a better mother and better wife. I wake up more alert and I sleep more soundly. I love knowing that I earned this new body. I am a whole new person and I feel so proud.*

• • • • •

Dana Davy-Bench, a married mother of two, was a member of Team Mallett even before Team Mallett existed. Nine months before Tracey's program began, Dana had been working out to Tracey's DVDs and lost a whopping 88 pounds. "Then I hit a plateau for a couple of months, so when I heard about Tracey's program I was excited to use her approach to lose the last of the weight," says this 27-year-old from Elk Grove, California.

Dana had struggled with her weight throughout her life, always carrying an extra 10–15 pounds on her 5-foot 2-inch frame. After having two children, that extra 15 pounds turned into an extra 75 pounds, and soon she tipped the scale at 200 pounds. "I would tell myself, 'You've had two kids in three years, you have a right to be fat,'" she says. "Obviously, I was in denial." All that changed one day when she caught a "devastating" glimpse of herself in the mirror and realized how big she had become. "I was so depressed and ashamed," says Dana. She jumped on the no-carb bandwagon and exercised on a treadmill. But she got minimal results and gave up when boredom set in. Then she discovered Tracey's workouts on *Exercise TV,* her cable provider's on-demand service, and began doing one workout five days a week. Instantly, she was hooked on Tracey's energetic, fun teaching style. "It was like having a trainer or friend working out with you. I lost weight immediately and began to love exercise," she says.

After Dana joined Team Mallett and began following the eating plan as well as the workouts, the pounds continued to come off. Dana saw her body tone up and noticed muscle definition from head to toe. "Exercise has become my thing. I have a real passion for working out and being in shape. It's part of who I am and something I really enjoy." Another thing that helped was that she could relate to Tracey. "She's also a mother of two young children and yet is in such great shape. Knowing that she's in the same boat I am made it seem all the more possible that I could do it, too," she says.

Changing her eating was the hardest part for Dana. "But what helped was Tracey's food journal," she says. Writing down what she ate and seeing it in front of her taught her about portion sizes and helped her make sure her diet was nutritionally balanced. "I realized that though I love food, it is *just* food. Now I think of it as fuel," she says. "You have to put the right amount and the right kind of fuel in your body to get the most out of your vehicle."

By the end of Tracey's six-week program, Dana weighed less than she did when she was a teenager. "I can't believe I turned my weight around. Two years ago I was a 5-foot 2-inch, 200-pound woman who wore a size 16. Today I weigh 113 pounds and wear a size 2," she says. The well-

DANA'S STICK-WITH-IT TIP

Know that you can do it. Realize that it takes work to lose weight and it's not always easy, but you can change your body into what you want it to be. Commit to it and realize that you're working toward being a healthier and stronger person.

deserved compliments have been pouring in. "I get so many compliments on how toned and in shape I am," she says. The best one is from her husband. "I had to tell him to stop calling me 'hot' so much because he was saying it ten times a day!" Best of all, Dana's life is better than ever—all thanks to her hard work and sweat. "Everything in my life is better since I lost the weight," she says. "My energy level is consistently high, my endurance is great. I love my body and truly feel proud about who I am now."

TRACEY'S TAKE

Where do I start? Dana is amazing, hard-working, and has extreme willpower. Every time I read her story I'm truly motivated to get my tennis shoes on. Exercise has empowered Dana to be the woman she's always wanted to be. She's now living her dream inside her dream body! What could be better than that?

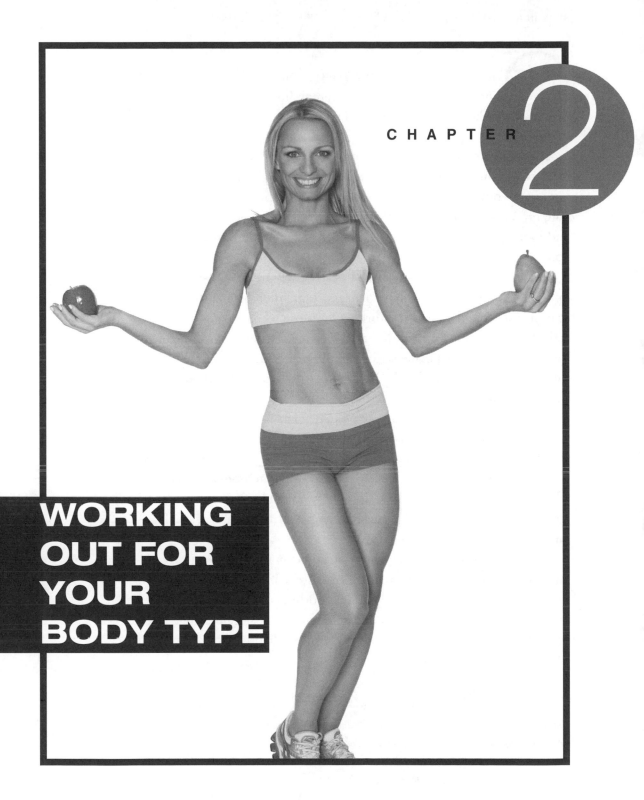

CHAPTER 2

WORKING
OUT FOR
YOUR
BODY TYPE

ONE OF THE MOST BEAUTIFUL THINGS ABOUT WOMEN'S bodies is that each one is different. Just take a glance around a locker room or beach and you'll know what I mean. The array of shapes and sizes is amazing. Still, most of us fall into one of two loose categories: apple or pear. I'm definitely a pear, which means I carry more weight in my lower body than my upper body. After years of working out, I know that I have to tailor my workout program to accommodate my smaller upper body and my ever-widening butt. Understanding and looking at your body will help you determine the best workout for you.

I've designed programs for two basic body types. I've also included options for women who want to focus more attention on a particular area as well as a general total-body workout for those who can't figure out exactly what's best for them. I loved the following comment from one of my Team Mallett members. She said, "I'm not one or the other, so I figured I'm a bowl of fruit and did the total-body conditioning workout." That was a good plan!

But regardless of your shape—apple, pear, or fruit salad—appreciate your body's strengths and make the most out of what you have. You can't alter your bone structure or change where your body naturally stores extra fat. Most of that is in our genes—a little gift from mom and dad. But what you *can* do is lose inches and tone your problem spots, which will give you a new sense of well-being and empowerment, as well as a fabulous figure, whatever its shape.

An easy way to see whether you're an apple or a pear is to start by taking a good look at your body in the mirror, preferably with no clothes on. Eyeball where most of your body fat is apportioned. (I'm sure you have a pretty good idea of this by now, but sometimes a pear can change to an apple after menopause, when you're more predisposed to abdominal

MOTIVATION FROM TEAM MALLETT

Exercise feels great; my body is changing, which feels awesome; and I want to keep going. The more I exercise, the easier it is, and it's good to feel and see the muscle tone.
—Robin Shaddy, 37, Papillon, Nebraska

fat.) The apple shape is medically known as an *android,* which in Greek means man. Gals with apple figures tend to have larger breasts, thin thighs, relatively no butt, and waists that are bigger than their hips. The pear is known as the *gynoid,* which is Greek for woman. Pear-shaped women usually have small waists and upper bodies and larger hips and butts. (Those with hourglass figures fit in the pear category, too.)

IDENTIFYING YOUR BODY SHAPE

You'll need a flexible tape-measure and a calculator.

- **Measure your middle.** Stand tall and try not to suck in your tummy. (I know it's tempting, but it won't help.) Then find your waist. If you have trouble finding it, look for the narrowest part of your midsection or find your belly button and use this as a marker. Take the measuring tape and put it around your waist. This measurement is your waist circumference.
- **Measure your hips.** Place the tape measure at least 3 to 4 inches below your belly button (the widest point of your hips and buttocks). This is your hip measurement.
- **Divide your waist circumference by your hip measurement.** This is your waist-to-hip ratio, which is also called your WHR.

You're a pear if your WHR is 0.80 or lower.
You're an apple if your WHR is higher than 0.80.

THE APPLE SHAPE

Apple-shaped gals typically gain weight around their middles. Fat around your middle—also known as a pot belly—often means you have visceral, or internal, fat that's surrounding your organs and sometimes even in the liver. We all have some visceral fat to protect our organs and act as an insulator. However, too much of this internal fat is not a good thing. It's more dangerous than carrying your weight around your booty, hips, and thighs like pears do because it can boost your blood sugar and increase your risk of heart disease, cancer, and diabetes. Research shows that these risks increase if your waist measurement is more than 35 inches. But you don't even have to have a major beer belly to have visceral fat. Even skinny-minnies with small pot bellies may have it. The key is to look at the waist-to-hip ratio: If the waist is wider than the hips, that could mean trouble.

Your genes are about 30 to 60 percent responsible for how much visceral fat you have. Some research has suggested that extra fat around the belly is also caused by a hormone called cortisol, which your body pumps out when under stress. At the same time, cortisol stimulates your cravings for fatty, sugar-filled foods. Foods that contain trans fats may also be to blame, suggests a study from Wake Forest University. This six-year study of monkeys found that those that ate trans fats increased their body weight by 7.2 percent while those that ate healthy monounsaturated fats (such as olive oil) had only a 1.8 percent increase. Even worse, the trans fat group had much bigger bellies by the end of the study than those eating the good-for-you fats. Although this was an animal study, it does suggest that, calorie for calorie, consuming trans fats leads to greater weight gain, especially in the belly area.

Enough of the bad news. The good news is that you can do something about this. Studies from Duke University Medical Center found that exercise can significantly reduce the amount of visceral fat clinging to an apple gal's tummy. Losing as little as 7 percent of your total body weight—just 10½ pounds on a 150-pound woman—can help. If, on the other hand, you keep your butt planted firmly on that couch, you'll not only pack on the pounds but also add more internal fat to your body. Another study in the *Journal of Applied Physiology* found that those who didn't exercise had an 8 percent increase in visceral fat in just six months. Yikes!

Apples usually have less muscle tone on their legs than on their upper body. Working the legs more frequently to build muscle mass and definition will balance the apple's appearance. Check out my *Sexy in 6* program suggestions for the typical apple on page 40.

WAIST CIRCUMFERENCE

Determine your waist circumference by placing a measuring tape snugly around your waist. If it's over 35 inches, this is a good indicator that you're carrying too much visceral fat.

TEAM MALLETT QUESTION

If I Work My Abs Every Day, Will It Burn the Fat Off My Abs?

Essentially, getting rid of body fat, and belly fat in particular, requires a whole-body approach. A common myth is that exercising the muscles beneath the fat on a certain body part will reduce that fat or that cutting out one group of "bad" foods will get the job done. Wrong. Fat loss occurs when the entire body is exercised and you're eating a healthy diet—exactly what you're doing when you follow *Sexy in 6*!

THE PEAR SHAPE

The pear shape, which means that you store most of your fat in the lower half of your body, is the most common shape for women. That's why many of us have that lovely area called saddlebags or—even worse—thunder thighs. Hourglass figures are also in this category. This fat is called subcutaneous fat, meaning it's fat just under the skin. (Who knew fat had so many different names?) This more superficial flab isn't as dangerous as the visceral fat, but often it's a lot more stubborn to get rid of. I can vouch for that!

As a pear shape, the hips, thighs, and butt may seem like a magnet for fat because gained weight may head straight to these areas. Genetically, this is your body's make-up, but my workouts will help minimize this. (What you can't change is your bone structure, such as naturally wide hips.) And of course, though you can change your shape with diet and exercise, you can't lengthen your legs (I wish!) or add inches to your height. I know some workouts advertise this, but let's just say that would be a miracle. What you can do is make your legs appear longer and leaner by doing the Quick Lower-Body Blast sculpting moves consistently.

Cellulite is usually an issue for us pear-shaped gals, thanks to the excess fat cells in this area. As women, we need this fat—lucky us—for child-bearing and breastfeeding years. (Ah, *that's* why you see so many more pear-shaped women than pear-shaped men!)

MOTIVATION FROM TEAM MALLETT

Two years ago, I was suffering from a very bad back condition that limited my activities. I started gaining weight rapidly for the first time in several years. To my dismay, all the weight went to my middle! I turned into the classic apple shape. With Tracey's plan of exercise and healthy eating, the weight left my midsection first! This allowed me to get back into clothes that I had been popping buttons on a few weeks before!
—Suanne Mendell, 60, La Canada, California

All-over strength training is essential for pears. The key is to increase your lean muscle mass and metabolic rate. Also, by building up the upper body and slimming the lower body, you can create the appearance of a more balanced figure. For maximum lower-body weight loss, I recommend bonus cardio (see page 177): spinning, cycling, hilly hikes, using the StairMaster, dancing, and kick boxing. They all work extremely well because their main focus is around the lower body.

Cross-training is the key to stimulating the lower body and not overusing the same muscles. One of the reasons why this plan works so well for pears is that each type of Quick Blast presents a different challenge, which keeps the body responding to the workouts. Switch Quick Blasts to avoid overusing the same muscles and prevent injury.

Check out the *Sexy in 6* typical pear program suggestions on page 41.

WHO KNEW?

Plus size sales are growing faster than size 10 and under. Despite our weight-obsessed society, half of all American women wear clothing in sizes 14 and larger.

TEAM MALLETT QUESTION

Will the StairMaster and Biking Make My Legs Too Big?
There's no way that you can build huge muscles performing high repetition with low intensity, even over a long period of time. To build muscle mass, you need to perform low repetition (6–8 reps) with heavy enough weights to go to fatigue. Regular cardiovascular exercise makes your legs toned, not overly muscled. Often after exercising, your legs may feel bigger. This is because when you work these muscles, they fill with blood and fluid, which gives you the feeling of them getting bigger. After a short time, they get back to normal. So calm down and hit the hills!

FIVE STEPS TO FREEDOM

1. Like yourself. Learn to accept the good with the bad. All of us have certain features we don't like but can't change. However, you can make these features look better through targeted exercises and a good diet. Growing up, I hated my legs and butt; I always felt they looked too masculine. It wasn't until I finally accepted that this was how they were and I was going to do the best I could with them that I finally liked them. Don't shy away from the mirror, look and find the parts of your body you like. Tell yourself repeatedly that you look hot.

2. Cop an attitude. If you put out positive energy, it will come back to you. If you want something, you will get it but only after you put your mind to it. Start this plan with the attitude that you're going to succeed. It sounds hard to believe, but I knew after the first week of the *Sexy in 6* program which members of Team Mallett would succeed. I could feel their energy and enthusiasm through their e-mails.

3. Step away from the scale. The worst thing you can do is constantly weigh yourself. I'll let you in on a little secret—there's no way you can put on pounds of fat overnight. To gain 1 pound, you would have to add 3,500 more calories to your normal diet. Now that's a lot of food! What are the chances of you eating 35 slices of bread? Not likely! There will be variations on the scale from morning to night just from the weight of food and water in your system. All that can make you weigh up to an extra 5 pounds. This is not fat, so don't stress or obsess over a number on a scale. The clothes test is much more accurate—if your clothes look good and you feel good, forget the numbers. Weigh yourself weekly or, better still, every other week. Choose the same time, preferably in the morning and midweek.

4. Don't give up. The reflection of your body on the outside is a true reflection of what is going on inside. I've watched clients curl up and cry when they stepped on the scale and saw that they were 2 pounds heavier. They just couldn't seem to get it into their heads that muscle weighs

TIPS FROM THE PROS: DRESS THE BEST FOR YOUR SHAPE

Carilyn Vaile, fashion designer and author of *I Am Diva! Every Woman's Guide to Outrageous Living,* has some simple tips for making your apple or pear look fabulous in clothes.

No tents! A large garment may be comfortable, but it is *never* flattering! Start experimenting with shapely silhouettes! If you have a smaller top and a larger bottom, wear blousy silhouettes (as opposed to fitted ones) with fitted skirts or straight-leg jeans and trousers.

Go all one color. If you're not ready to take risks playing with color, dress in one color. This elongates the look of your body.

more than fat or that they could be carrying excess water. Then they usually binged on food for comfort instead of thinking about how they really feel. Before clients get on the scale, I ask them to give me an unbiased comment on how they feel about their body. Then if their weight is not what they expected, I'll gently remind them of what they've just told me. It can work both ways; sometimes clients feel like they haven't accomplished anything, and then they get on the scale and see that it's not that bad. It's always a big surprise.

5. Have fun. Laugh and pretend that you enjoy exercising. You may surprise yourself and have fun. An optimistic attitude goes a long way.

LEARN TO ACCEPT COMPLIMENTS

When the compliments about your new body and gorgeous glow start pouring in, accept them! Most women aren't good at this. We can dole out compliments to our friends, our kids, and the barista at Starbucks, but when *we* get a little praise we refute it. Usually it goes something like this: You're at the mall when you run into a friend you haven't seen in a few months. She says, "Wow, Joanna, you look great. Look how toned your arms are!" Before she can finish her sentence, you're saying, "But they're still flabby and I've got a few pounds to lose off my butt." All of a sudden you've nixed everything your friend has said. You haven't even heard her compliment because you've been so busy filling the air with negative words about yourself.

Next time, think of it this way: A compliment is a gift the other person is giving you. Now you wouldn't open a gift and then immediately shove it back in your friend's hand, saying, "I don't want this." Well, that's exactly what you're doing when you dispute a compliment. Instead, say, "Thank you" and shut up. Literally bite your tongue if you must, but let those positive words linger in the air. Let them soak in. You deserve it!

MOTIVATION FROM TEAM MALLETT

I was shocked at the changes in my body after just two weeks.
I lost an inch in my waist, hips, and thighs!
—Liz Price, 37, South Pasadena, California

CALCULATING YOUR BMI

HOW TO CALCULATE YOUR BMI

MEASUREMENT UNITS
Formula and Calculation

KILOGRAMS AND METERS (or centimeters)

Formula: weight (kg) / [height (m)]^2

With the metric system, the formula for BMI is weight in kilograms divided by height in meters squared.
Since height is commonly measured in centimeters, divide height in centimeters by 100 to obtain height in meters.

Example: Weight = 68 kg, Height = 165 cm (1.65 m)
Calculation: 68 ÷ (1.65)^2 = 24.98

POUNDS AND INCHES

Formula: weight (lb) / [height (in)]^2 x 703

Calculate BMI by dividing weight in pounds (lbs) by height in inches (in) squared and multiplying by a conversion factor of 703.

Example: Weight = 150 lbs, Height = 5'5" (65 inches)
Calculation: [150 ÷ (65)^2] x 703 = 24.96

Source: Centers for Disease Control.

CLASSIFICATION OF OVERWEIGHT AND OBESITY BY BMI, WAIST CIRCUMFERENCE, AND ASSOCIATED DISEASE RISKS

	BMI (kg/m^2)	OBESITY CLASS	DISEASE RISK* RELATIVE TO NORMAL WEIGHT & WAIST CIRCUMFERENCE	
			WOMEN 88 cm (35 in) OR LESS	WOMEN > 88 cm (35 in)
Underweight	< 18.5		–	–
Normal	18.5–24.9		–	–
Overweight	25.0–29.9		Increased	High
Obesity	30.0–34.9	I	High	Very High
	35.0–39.9	II	Very High	Very High
Extreme Obesity	40.0†	III	Extremely High	Extremely High

*Disease risk for type 2 diabetes, hypertension, and CVD.
†Increased waist circumference can also be a marker for increased risk even in persons of normal weight.

Source: Department of Health and Human Services

Your body mass index, or BMI, is a measurement of your weight based on your height. The CDC (Centers for Disease Control) says it's the best method for predicting obesity and health concerns (much more so than just weight). Women tend to have a higher BMI than men because we carry more body fat. (As mentioned, extra fat storage is essential for child rearing and breastfeeding.) One of the major drawbacks of the BMI is that it doesn't take into account people who have a high amount of lean muscle mass. Muscle is denser than fat, so it weighs more. So make sure you take that into consideration when you calculate your BMI. (Muscle also takes up less space than fat, so you can weigh the same but wear a smaller dress size. I'll take that any day!)

Success Story

Emily Cole, 28, single mother of two, Fort Worth, Texas

Lost

9 pounds

Two dress sizes

2 inches off her waist

3 inches off her hips

2 inches off her legs

7 inches total

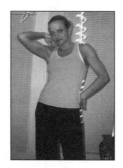
Before

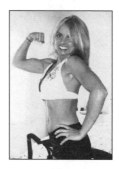
After

Gained

Her self-esteem. *I have newfound confidence! Being divorced with two young kids can really hurt your self-image. However, now that I'm back in shape, I feel fantastic! Being fit truly is a natural antidepressant!*

• • • • •

To say Emily Cole, 28, has a hectic life is an understatement. She's a single mother of two toddlers who was working full time and going to school full time when she joined Team Mallett. Although Emily had never been heavy as a child or a teen, she now carried extra pounds on her 5-foot 3-inch frame. "I'd gotten married and I let myself go," she says. "The weight made me feel disgusting, lazy, and uncomfortable, both mentally and physically."

Every now and then she'd try exercising but would get bored and give up. Before joining Team Mallett, Emily was jogging for thirty minutes during lunch but didn't have the time to do much more. The processed high-carb sugary foods that filled her diet, such as Pop-Tarts, TV dinners, and "anything fast and in a box," didn't help either. After she began the program, though, her sweet tooth subsided. "I've always struggled with cravings for sugary treats. Once I started following Tracey's workout and felt like I was getting into shape, however, I didn't want these foods half as much," she says.

After just a few weeks, Emily noticed more tone and definition in her body—especially her arms and shoulders—and friends were telling her that she'd lost weight. She realized that just because she couldn't make it to the gym didn't mean she couldn't be fit and active. She worked hard to be consistent despite "the daily hardballs of life that kept coming my way!" She says, "I still wake up every morning at 5 and do my workout." In fact, her chaotic life is one reason Emily loves Tracey's workouts. "They have inspired me and opened a whole new world of fitness for me. I've always worked out in a gym, but working out from home is just as effective while saving me lots of time and money. Plus, it is more convenient since I can do it at 2:00 A.M. if I want to. That works wonderfully with my schedule and doesn't take time away from my children."

Exercising regularly and eating right weren't the only healthy changes Emily made. She also quit smoking and realized that exercise could help her relieve some of the stress from her busy life as a working, single mom. Six weeks into the program, she was thrilled when a size four pair of jeans from high school fit. "I'm in better shape now than when I was 16 years old and a track star! I have even more definition in my abs, and my butt is sticking out just a bit more—in a good way!" But the benefits for Emily go way beyond looking fabulous in jeans from her teen years. "This whole program has changed my life and put me back on the road

EMILY'S STICK-WITH-IT TIP

Think of working out as the foundation for a better way of living. When you work out, it helps your body crave healthy foods and motivates you to not want to counteract all the work you've just done!

to good health. I have more energy. But most of all, I feel strong and confident!"

TRACEY'S TAKE

From the first e-mail I received from Emily, I was blown away by her energy; it just bounced off the computer screen. Wow, I thought, this is my kind of gal! She's such an inspiration to all those women with children who say, "I don't have enough time." Emily's life is stressful—to say the least! She's bringing up two children on her own, working, and going back to school. All that leaves her feeling exhausted. In the past, she would start to work out, and then a stressful situation would arise and she would eat to solve the problem. What she's learned is how exercise can help with the effects of stress and give her more energy to focus on herself. She deserves it!

MOTIVATION FROM TEAM MALLETT

I had been doing spin classes four to five times per week for more than a year, but I still struggled with a flabby stomach and oversize hips. In just four weeks on Tracey's plan, I can see a difference in both my abs and hips, and I couldn't be more thrilled. I have struggled with both areas all my adult life, so it feels great to finally see a positive change! I will continue these workouts forever.
—Loren Alison, 47, South Pasadena, California

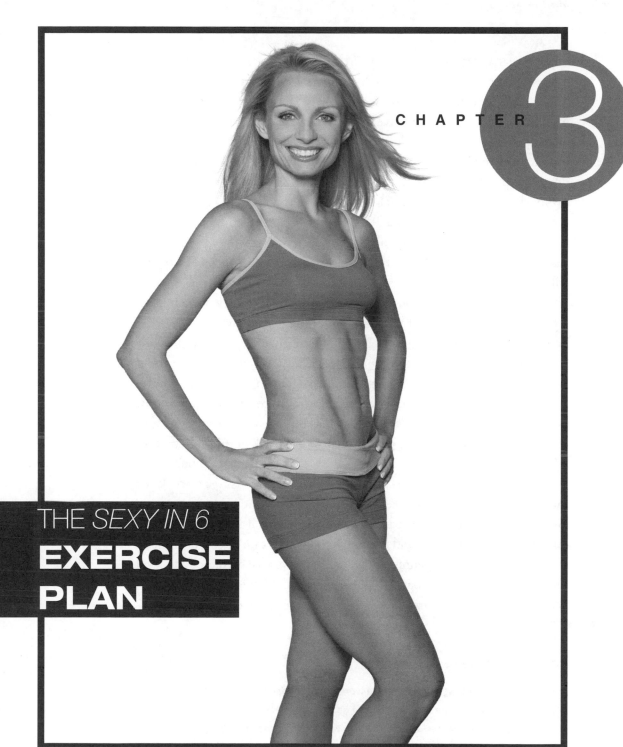

CHAPTER 3

THE *SEXY IN 6*
**EXERCISE
PLAN**

A S WOMEN, WE'RE NATURAL MULTITASKERS. JUGGLING A million things at the same time is second nature to us. And if the truth be known, we probably wouldn't have it any other way. Between being a taxi driver for my kids, teaching classes, training clients, working on this book, and being married, my life is chaos. But it's fun chaos. It makes life worth living. Still, there are days I'd like to slow down, stop looking at my watch, and live without a schedule. But that's in my dreams, so I have to get real. The only way to get real when it comes to fitness is finding small increments of time throughout the day to squeeze it in. People always ask me my secret for staying in shape, and that's it. Not much of a secret, but it works! That's why the *Sexy in 6* plan will work for you, too.

All the plans are eighteen minutes a day, six days a week, for a total of six weeks. They consist of three six-minute segments, which can easily be spread throughout the day or done all at once depending on your schedule. The *Sexy in 6* six-minute Quick Blasts consist of deep-toning and fat-burning techniques from Pilates, yoga, weight training, sports conditioning, kick boxing, and dance. Because we're all made differently, the plan allows you to customize the workout for your body type and goals. It's as simple as identifying your workout track in this chapter and following it consistently for six weeks. Now how hard can that be?

Optional bonus cardio is suggested two to three times a week for those who want maximum calorie burn. I've even included six-minute interval Cardio Blasts to get you started. However, if finding that extra time is simply impossible and too much to incorporate into your lifestyle at this moment, grab a pedometer and start to increase your activity level throughout the day (see page 184). Or better still, have some fun underneath the sheets! Sex burns lots of calories—check out chapter 9.

MOTIVATION FROM TEAM MALLETT

Participating in your program has been a wonderful experience.
What I love the most about it is that you can get a great workout
in a very short period of time and feel like you've accomplished something.
—Laurie Jardin, 43, Ontario, Canada

Following is a Team Mallett member's schedule. (See Appendix A for a workout log of your own.) Debbie is a working mom whose goal is general total-body conditioning. She found that she could easily fit in twelve to eighteen minutes of exercise in the morning before she went to work. She was surprised to find that it gave her more energy to tear through her to do-list and other obligations. It also set a healthy tone for the day. Exercising in the evening was a struggle for her because she felt guilty taking time for herself. After all, she'd been at work all day and wanted to be with her kids—plus she had to squeeze in homework help, making dinner, and bath time. However, finding six minutes wasn't hard for her. Some nights she'd do the moves while helping her kids with homework. They got used to mom lunging as they did long division and squatting while she quizzed them on their weekly spelling words. Other nights, the kids would join her in her workouts and the giggles were nonstop. Thursday night was her cardio night, so she made sure her husband got home early enough to take over childcare and let her break her sweat solo.

Tracey's Tips

• Photocopy your workout plan exercises and staple them together so they're easily accessible and organized.
• If you find yourself with more time on your hands and want to fit in another segment, fire away! On the other hand, if you're having a busy day and can fit in only a couple of Blasts, that's fine; just try and make up the other Blasts during the rest of the week.

DEBBIE'S TEAM MALLETT WORKOUT

	MON	TUES	WED	THUR	FRI	SAT
6 am	Total Body Blast A & B (12 mins)	Mind Body Blast A & B (12 mins) Upper Body Blast A (6 mins)	Lower Body Blast A & B (12 mins)	Total Blast A, B & C (18 minutes)	Upper Body Blast B & C (12 mins)	Lower Body Blast B & C (12 mins)
Lunch						Quick Abs Blast A (6 mins)
PM	Abs Blast A (6 mins)		Abs Blast B (6 mins)		Mind Body Blast C (6 mins)	

Now it's your turn to find your body type or your personal goal program and stick to that plan.

GENERAL TOTAL-BODY CONDITIONING

Do you just want general total-body conditioning? If so, here's your workout.

WORKOUT FOR GENERAL TOTAL-BODY CONDITIONING

MON	TUES	WED	THUR	FRI	SAT	SUN
Total Body Blast A & B	Mind Body Blast A & B	Total Body Blast A & C	Lower Body Blast A, B & C	Upper Body Blast B & C	Lower Body Blast B & C	Day Off
Abs Blast A	Upper Body Blast A	Abs Blast B		Mind Body Blast C	Abs Blast A	

WORKOUT FOR APPLES

Are you a classic apple who carries more weight around your midsection? Your workout focuses on overall toning for weight loss with an emphasis on building strength and tone in your legs. The latter helps balance the proportions of an apple-shaped body. As I mentioned in chapter 2, stress releases a hormone called cortisol that is believed to increase the fat that apples carry around their bellies. Doing a regular mind-body practice helps reduce stress. Also, the added toning from Pilates for the core is essential to whittling your middle and helping support the spine that's carrying excess torso weight.

WORKOUT FOR APPLES

MON	TUES	WED	THUR	FRI	SAT	SUN
Total Body Blast A & B	Lower Body Blast A & B	Mind Body Blast A & B	Total Body Blast B & C	Mind Body Blast B & C	Lower Body Blast B & C	Day Off
Abs Blast A	Abs Blast B	Upper Body Blast A	Abs Blast A	Upper Body Blast B	Abs Blast B	

WORKOUT FOR PEARS

If you're a classic pear and want to reduce the excess weight in your lower body, start by following the plan in this section. For further weight loss, try six-minute interval training workouts (see workout suggestions in chapter 8) and progress to longer sessions as you feel stronger. Incorporating short higher-intensity intervals into your plan will help expedite the release of that stubborn lower-body fat. Unfortunately, most pears usually lose their upper-body fat deposits first. But by consistently doing the Quick Total and Lower-Body Blasts, you force your body to take fat from the lower body. (Isn't that exciting?)

Interval training is when you vary the intensity of your workout between very intense and moderate. For example, you might run at your fastest pace (around 7.0 mph) for one minute and then walk at 4.5 mph for two minutes, alternating like this for the duration of your workout. Interval training burns more calories than exercising at one steady pace, and it's one of the reasons why I've worked small intervals into most of my workouts. Interval training is also a good way to squeeze an effective workout into a short period of time. In other words, if you have limited time and want to burn the most calories, do short higher-intensity intervals throughout your workout. For example, when running or walking, incorporate some hills and climb them as fast as you can, elevating you heart rate until you probably can say only about ten to fifteen words per thirty seconds. Or try my downloadable workouts at iamplify.com. (Look at Appendix C for more information and how to get a discount.)

Tracey's Tip

Don't make the mistake of eating more to compensate for working out more!

WORKOUT FOR PEARS						
MON	TUES	WED	THUR	FRI	SAT	SUN
Total Body Blast A & B	Lower Body Blast A & B	Total Body Blast B & C	Mind Body Blast A & C	Lower Body Blast A & C	Total Body Blast A & C	Day Off
Upper Body Blast A	Abs Blast A	Abs Blast B	Upper Body Blast B	Abs Blast B	Upper Body Blast C	

THE ABS AND BUTT WORKOUT

Do you want to get rid of your tummy and perk up your butt? Here's your plan.

WORKOUT FOR ABS AND BUTT

MON	TUES	WED	THUR	FRI	SAT	SUN
Total Body Blast A, B & C	Lower Body Blast B & C	Total Body Blast A & B	Lower Body Blast A & B	Total Body Blast A & B	Mind Body Blast B & C	Day Off
	Upper Body Blast A	Abs Blast B	Abs Blast A	Abs Blast B	Upper Body Blast B	

THE ARMS AND ALL-OVER BODY WORKOUT

Do you want to focus more on your arms with general all-over body conditioning? Here's your plan.

WORKOUT FOR ARMS AND ALL OVER BODY

MON	TUES	WED	THUR	FRI	SAT	SUN
Total Body Blast A & B	Upper Body Blast A & B	Total Body Blast A & B	Upper Body Blast C & D	Lower Body Blast A & B	Upper Body Blast A & B	Day Off
Abs Blast A	Lower Body Blast A	Abs Blast B	Lower Body Blast B	Mind Body Blast A	Abs Blast A	

QUICK UPPER-BODY BLAST A

A quick reference guide. For more information on the exercises, see page 65.

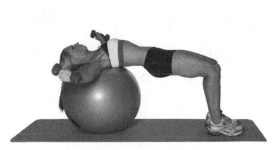

1. BRIDGE FLY

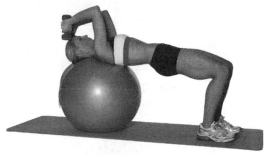

2. BRIDGE TRICEP EXTENSION

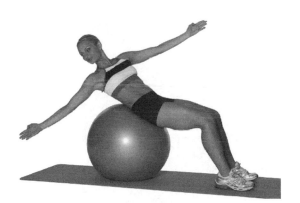

3. ABDOMINAL ROLL WITH REACH

TIPS FROM THE PROS

"A fitness routine is a good idea for everyone, but for those with digestive issues, such as indigestion, heartburn, constipation, ulcerative colitis, or irritable bowel syndrome, it's especially helpful," says Elizabeth Lipski, Ph.D., CCN, author of *Digestive Wellness*. "Exercise increases circulation while massaging and toning your entire digestive system."

QUICK UPPER-BODY BLAST B

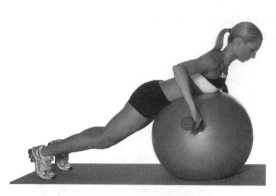

1. ROW ON THE BALL

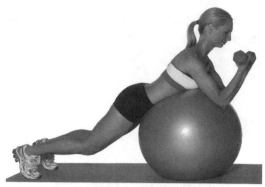

2. PREACHER CURLS

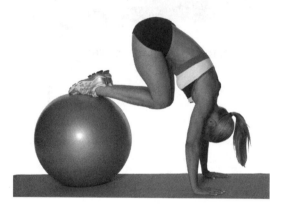

3. RABBIT ON THE BALL

MOTIVATION FROM TEAM MALLETT

I enjoy the Sexy in 6 exercises because they're so different and there's so much variety in a short workout. It isn't just straight sit-ups, lunges, and squats, which can become really boring. I love the inclusion of the dance movements and the sequence building.
—Sue Guidice, 50, Perth, Australia

QUICK UPPER-BODY BLAST C

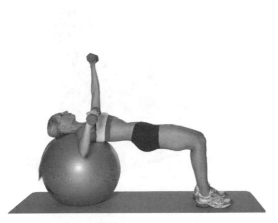

1. SINGLE-ARM CHEST PRESS

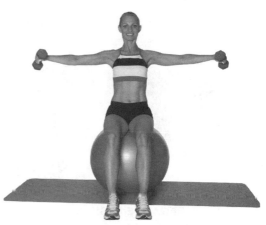

2. LATERAL RAISES

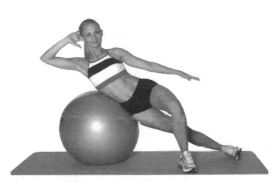

3. SIDE-OVERS

MOTIVATION FROM TEAM MALLETT

I'm feeling good and I love my increased energy level. This plan is good for new moms like me, because it allows you to get in a workout here and there when you don't have hours to spend at the gym. The workouts have been short, sweet, and to the point—I love it!
—Stephanie Fleig, 26, Arkansas City, Kansas

QUICK UPPER-BODY BLAST D

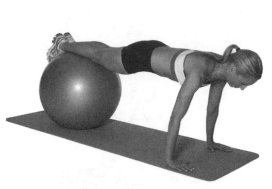

1. NEGATIVE PUSH-UPS

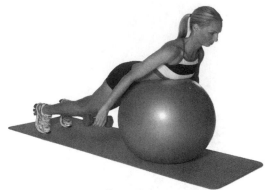

2. LAT PULL

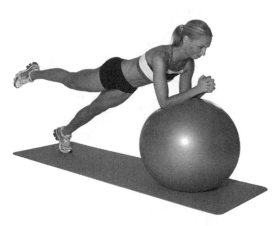

3. FOREARM ELBOW BALANCE

MOTIVATION FROM TEAM MALLETT

The twelve-minute workouts are great—absolutely something I can fit in with family and kids when they are sleeping in the morning. Or if they're up, they can jump around with me for twelve minutes without getting too ridiculously bored.
— Erin Lamb, 37, San Marino, California

SHORT AND SWEET STRETCHES

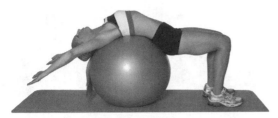

1. BACK STRETCH

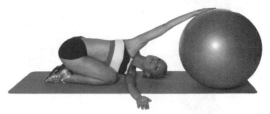

2. THREADING THE NEEDLE

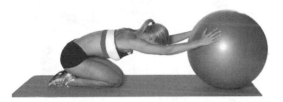

3. CHILD'S POSE

QUICK LOWER-BODY BLAST A

A quick reference guide. For more information on the exercises, see page 90.

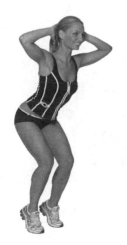

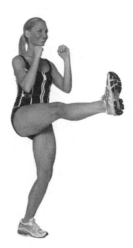

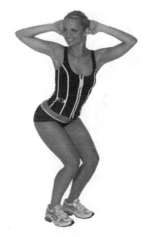

**1. TRAVELING SIDE SQUATS
ON TOES**

2. KICK SQUATS

**3. THIRTY-SECOND INTERVAL:
JUMP SQUAT TWIST**

QUICK LOWER-BODY BLAST B

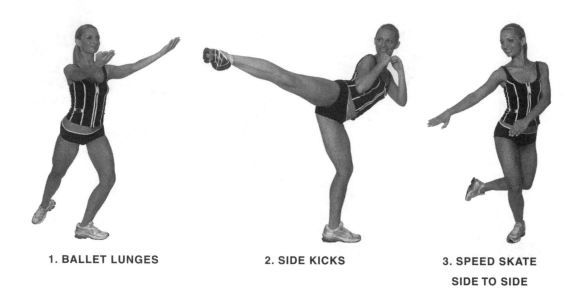

1. BALLET LUNGES

2. SIDE KICKS

3. SPEED SKATE
SIDE TO SIDE

QUICK LOWER-BODY BLAST C

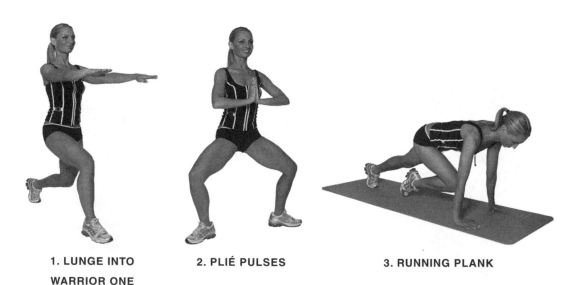

1. LUNGE INTO
WARRIOR ONE

2. PLIÉ PULSES

3. RUNNING PLANK

STRETCHES

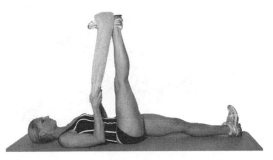

1. HAMSTRING STRETCH WITH TOWEL

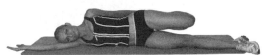

2. QUAD STRETCH

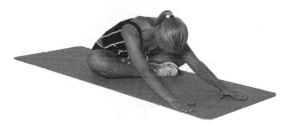

3. SITTING CROSS-LEG STRETCH

QUICK ABS BLAST A

A quick reference guide. For more information on the exercises, see page 113.

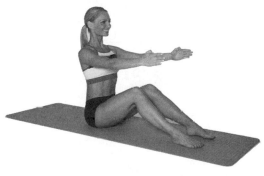

1. CIRCLE ROLL-UP

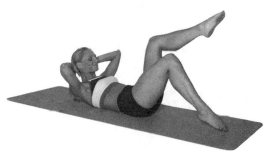

2. DIPPING THE TOES

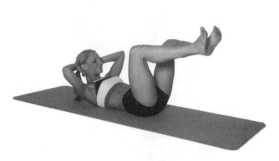

3. FROGGIES

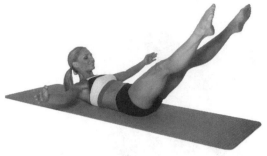

4. ABDOMINAL OPENINGS

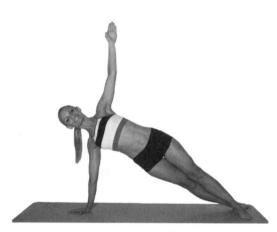

5. SIDE PLANK TWIST

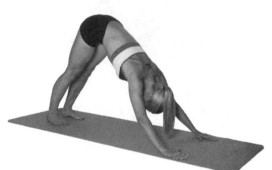

6. PLANK TO DOWNWARD DOG

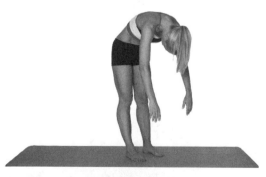

7. ROLL-DOWN

QUICK ABS BLAST B ON THE BALL

A quick reference guide. For more information on the exercises, see page 121.

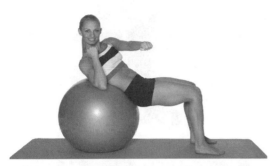

1. JAB CROSS ON THE BALL

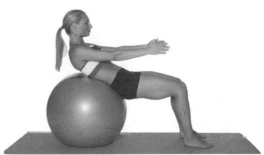

2. CHEST LIFT WITH ARM REACH

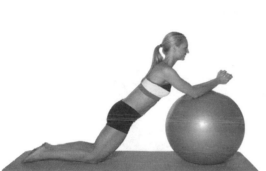

3. DOWN STRETCH

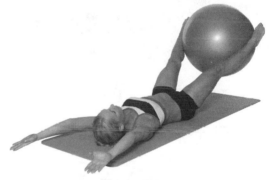

4. BALL SWITCH

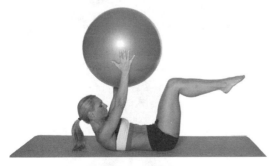

5. CLASSIC DOUBLE LEG STRETCH

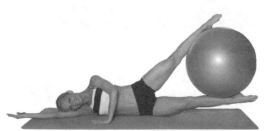

6. DOUBLE LEG SIDE LIFTS

QUICK MIND-BODY BLAST A

A quick reference guide. For more information on the exercises, see page 134.

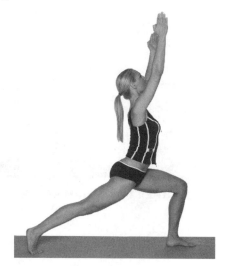

1. CRESCENT LUNGE

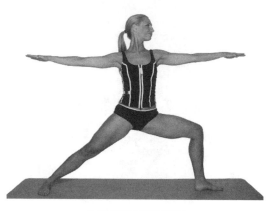

2. WARRIOR TWO

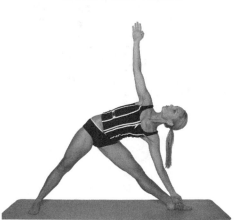

3. TRIANGLE POSE

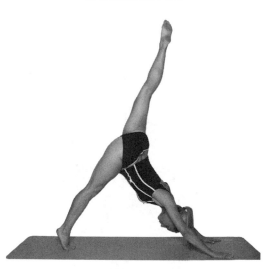

4. DOG SPLITS

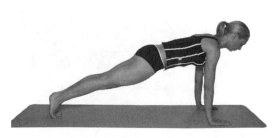

5. PLANK POSITION

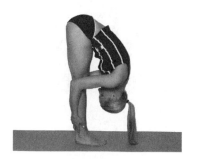

6. STANDING HEAD-TO-KNEE

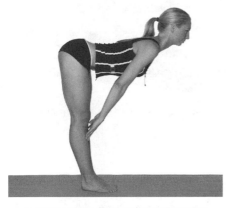

7. STANDING SPINE EXTENSION

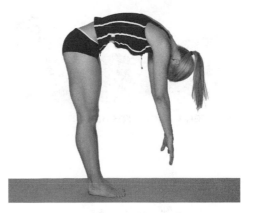

8. ROLL-UP

QUICK MIND-BODY BLAST B

A quick reference guide. For more information on these 5 exercises, see page 140.

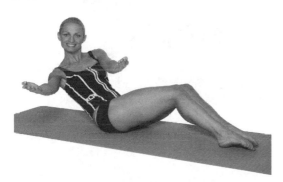

1. KNEE TWISTS

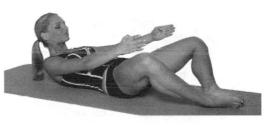

2. CHEST LIFT WITH ARM REACH IN BUTTERFLY POSITION

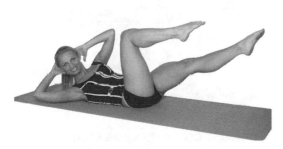

3. SINGLE LEG STRETCH INTO CRISS-CROSS

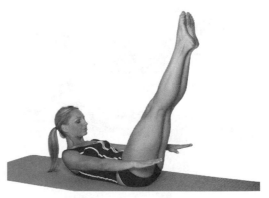

4. DOUBLE LEG STRETCH

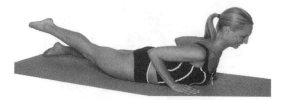

5. FLUTTER KICKS WITH HEEL BEATS

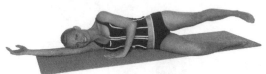

6. PILATES SIDE LEG SERIES

QUICK MIND-BODY BLAST C

A quick reference guide. For more information on the exercises, see page 147.

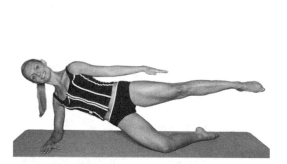

1. SIDE PLANK LEG LIFT

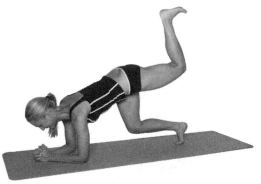

2. DOLPHIN KICK BACKS

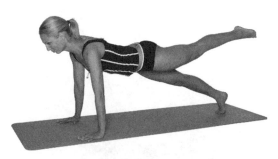

3. LEG PULL FRONT

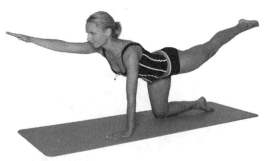

4. CAT COW WITH LEG EXTENSION

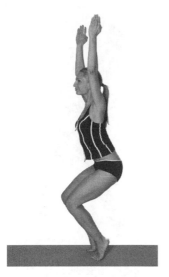

**5. CHAIR POSITION WITH
HEELS ELEVATED**

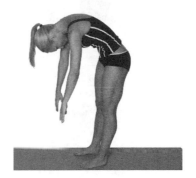

6. ROLL-DOWN

QUICK CARDIO BLAST A

A quick reference guide. For more information on the exercises, see
page 165.

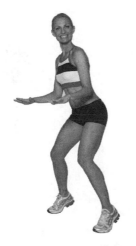

1. BOUNCING BALL SHUFFLE

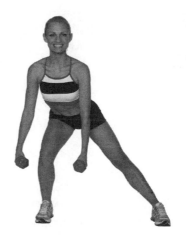

2. SIDE LUNGE WITH ROW

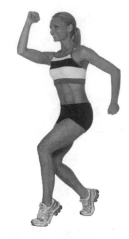

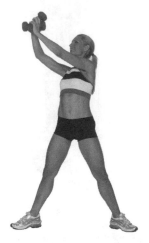

3. ONE-MINUTE INTERVAL:

SPLIT LUNGE CROSS COUNTRY

4. CHOPPING WOOD

QUICK CARDIO BLAST B

A quick reference guide. For more information on the exercises, see page 169.

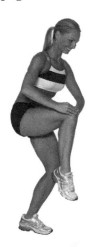

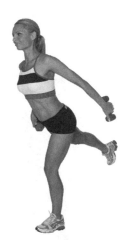

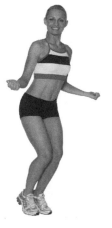

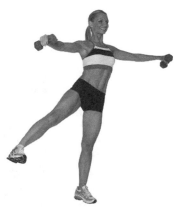

1. KNEE
REPEATER
AB CRUNCH

2. HAMSTRING
CURLS WITH
TRICEPS EXTENSIONS

3. ONE-MINUTE
INTERVAL:
PRETEND TO
SKIP ROPE

4. SQUAT LIFT
WITH LATERAL
SIDE LIFTS

QUICK CARDIO BLAST C

A quick reference guide. For more information on the exercises, see page 173.

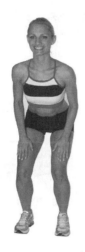 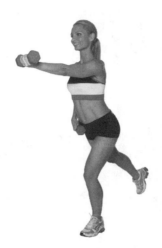 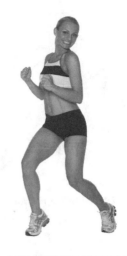

1. DOUBLE PULSE SQUATS WITH JUMP

2. FLAMINGO WITH BICEPS LIFT

3. ONE-MINUTE INTERVAL: CHUGGA, CHOO, CHOO

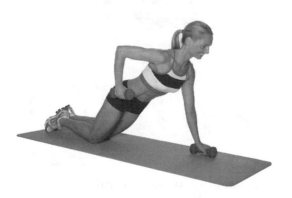

4. PLANK WITH ROW

CARDIO STRETCHES

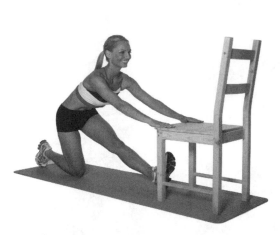

1. LUNGE INTO HAMSTRING STRETCH

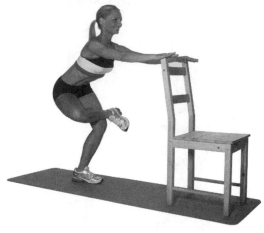

2. FIGURE-FOUR HIP STRETCH

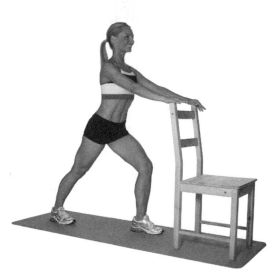

3. CALF STRETCH

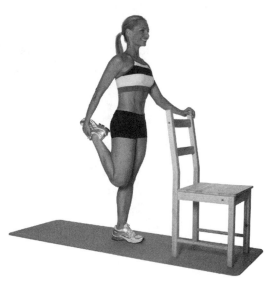

4. QUAD STRETCH

MOTIVATION FROM TEAM MALLETT

I've lost 16 pounds in 6 weeks and couldn't believe that I put on a suit from just a couple of months before the program and my husband told me to take it off because it was way too big, I was so happy to hear that!
—Niki Robinson, 33, Fayetteville, Georgia

Success Story

Lynn Serwin, 45, mother of twins, South Pasadena, California

Lost

15 pounds

Two dress sizes

2 inches off her chest

1 inch off her arms

2 inches off her waist

2½ inches off her hips

7½ inches total

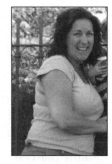
Before

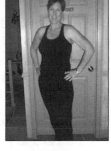
After

Gained

A can-do attitude and a body that I'm comfortable with. *I'm more positive than ever after succeeding on this program, I know now that I can achieve whatever I want and that's very empowering.*

• • • • •

Lynne Serwin, 45, had always been an overeater, using food as a response to both the good and bad times in her life. Overeating made her feel better for a short period of time but soon she'd feel worse than before. For most of Lynn's life she carried an extra 40 pounds and was borderline obese. To make matters worse, when she got pregnant five years ago, she gained 70 extra pounds. "I was very dissatisfied with my body image and felt unattractive and depressed. I wanted to stop losing and gaining that same 20 pounds," says the school teacher. It wasn't until she joined Team Mallett that Lynn got results.

LYNN'S STICK-WITH-IT TIP

Even if you don't feel like exercising, do it everyday.
It only takes a few minutes and the benefits to your fitness, energy,
and emotional well-being are well worth spending the time.

One reason she went on the plan was to learn healthy eating habits. Before, Lynn ate a breakfast of bran cereal, yogurt with fruit and smoothies but any positive effects were cancelled by the pizza and fried food she ate for lunch and dinner. Snacks included ice cream, cookies and cakes. She was clueless about healthy cooking and portion sizes. Lynn was pleasantly surprised by Tracey's food plan. "I realized there are healthy foods that taste wonderful," she says. "I am rarely hungry because I eat smaller portions more often, and I have learned not to eat huge portions. Understanding how nutrition works and knowing that I'm not deprived, but rather motivated, by my success keeps me sticking to the food plan."

In her pre-Team Mallett days, Lynn's exercise routine consisted of doing cardio and Pilates, which wasn't giving her the results she longed for. However Tracey's DVD and easy-to-follow plan changed her thinking on exercise, too. "Tracey's program made me realize that you can get results in short amounts of time working out in little increments throughout the day. It's a fun way to stay healthy and feel great," she says. Of course there were times when she was tired and "just wanted to lie down," but Lynn focused on the great feeling she had when she finished a workout. She also stayed motivated knowing she would see results if she stuck with it, and she was right. Just four weeks into the program, Lynn shed pounds and found that her clothes were much looser.

Today, fifteen pounds lighter than when she started, Lynn feels better than ever and says she's light on her feet and energized. "I sleep better, I walk faster and I have extra energy to play with my 5-year-old twins," she says. "I'm not winded after walking up a flight of stairs. The mental benefits are equally as satisfying. I'm more alert and positive. Now I want to exercise and eat right, which is a life-altering mind set. This program is the best thing that's happened to me in a long time."

TRACEY'S TAKE

Lynn reached a goal that she originally thought was impossible and along the way she realized that exercising is fun. She no longer viewed it as a chore. The good results kept her going until finally it became a good habit. Once anyone gets to this point there's no looking back; you've tasted the good life and you feel on fire! Lynn is exactly that. She's on fire and ready to keep on exercising for life!

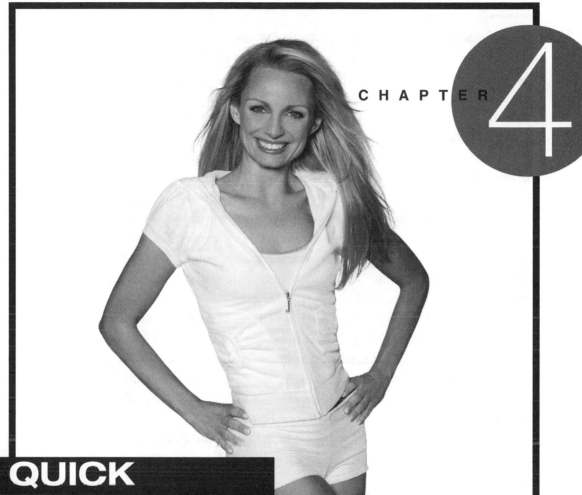

CHAPTER 4

QUICK
UPPER-BODY
BLAST

EVEN IF YOU AREN'T A CELEBRITY WATCHER OR DON'T GIVE A hoot about Hollywood's A-list, you have to admit that some of the arms, shoulders, and backs you see on the red carpet, on TV, or in the movies are sexy. Think Jennifer Aniston, Angela Bassett, Sheryl Crow. They're toned and sculpted, and they can easily wear upper-body-baring fashions without thinking twice. There's nothing more elegant than beautiful biceps or shoulders peeking out from beneath a tank top or strapless gown.

On the flip side, there's nothing scarier than a ripple of flab dangling from below your upper arms, jiggling as you wave good-bye. And just when you thought it couldn't get any worse, there's bra fat! Yes, there's actually a *name* for that bulge spilling over the back of your bra strap. But if those images don't do it for you, here's a horror story that will have you running for your dumbbells.

I had a client who I'll call Melissa. It was a hot summer day and she was at a family reunion, sitting there with an endless stream of relatives, including all the nieces and nephews. She was wearing a tank top. Well, her 4-year-old niece came up to her, jiggled the flesh beneath her upper arm, and said, "Aunt Melissa, this looks just like the turkey we saw at the zoo yesterday!" Out of the mouths of babes! Her niece was excited by the comparison, but Melissa was mortified. She called me up the next day in tears. From then on, she worked harder on her arms than any other client I've ever had.

This story even scared *me* into putting a little more effort into my upper body. But the true beauty of working your arms, shoulders, chest, and back is that it makes you strong. And when you're strong, life is just a whole lot easier. It makes carrying your kids, briefcase, and groceries easier. You no longer have to ask your husband to lift stuff for you (or get annoyed that he's not doing it) or have that teenage cashier at the grocery store carry your bags to your car. Think of the tips you'll save! (And you can always fake it when that hunky guy happens to be around.)

So with all this, why do lots of women avoid working their upper body? Two words: Linda Hamilton. Remember her man-like, super-carved arms in *Terminator?* Her biceps almost rivaled Arnold Schwarzenegger's! I loved the strong woman she portrayed, but her arms made many of my female clients drop their weights like hot potatoes. They were filled with a fear of bulking up. The truth is there's just no way that most women can get big, super-cut arms. The reason men get all that muscle is because of all their testosterone. We have some of that hormone in our bodies, but not nearly as much as they do. Trust me, women just can't get there. The female body-builders you see on TV or in magazines eat a huge amount of protein and work out 24/7—it's their life! Now if you have that much time on your hands, put this book down because you certainly don't need *Sexy in 6!*

One client of mine was so paranoid about her arms getting too big that, even after a year of weight training, she'd only use 5-pound dumbbells for biceps curls. She was standing next to this huge body-builder and thought she was going to end up looking like him. I kept telling her, "Don't be scared!" Think about it. If we could bulk up that much or that quickly, we'd barely have to exercise our arms at all. So forget the fear (or that excuse). This goes for all body parts. Even if you are one of the rare women with the genetics to get that way, you'll know it pretty quickly.

The workouts in this chapter will make your arms lean, elegant, and toned. We're going for endurance using light weights and doing two sets of 10–15 reps. By building muscle, you'll boost your metabolism. And by boosting your metabolism, you'll burn more overall body fat.

Another thing many women don't realize is that you can't just do a few bicep curls and triceps extensions, call it a day, and hope to have sleek, sexy arms. Nope. Sorry. The upper body should have a nice symmetrical and balanced look. Remember that song from grade school: "The hip bone is connected to the knee bone. The knee bone is connected to the shin bone"? The same goes for all those upper-body muscles. If you want lean, toned arms, you've actually got to work the chest, back, and shoulders, too. For example, you know that sexy little indented V in the upper arms? Well, that's not the result of just doing bicep curls. It's from doing a well-balanced upper-body program.

At this point, maybe a light bulb is going off and you're realizing why, after years of doing random arm exercises once in a while, your arms are more sausage-like than sleek. The good news is that you don't have to work your arms long and hard to get results. You'll see that from the six-minute upper-body workouts! These are the exercises I do about twice a week. I hate working my upper body, so I've created a program that gets me in and out of that body part fast with results. This plan will also help you shed fat to make your arms look good. After all, what's the point of sexy, sculpted muscles if they're hidden under a layer of flab?

Another less exciting reason to exercise *all* the muscles of your upper body is to prevent injuries. For example, if you buff up your shoulders and biceps but neglect to work your small rotator cuff muscles (those that hold your shoulder joint in place), they'll get weak. Eventually those lazy bums will stop doing their job, causing your poor old biceps and deltoids (shoulders) to work overtime. Eventually, this imbalance can cause injury—and pain! Lots of it.

Unfortunately, I know this firsthand. (Yes, me! Someone who exercises for her day job!) I've spent the last five years picking up my kids with one arm (also not advised). Sure, from that alone I now have strong deltoids and biceps. But since then, I was a bad girl and didn't work my rotator cuffs. I thought, hey, they're not visible, so why spend the time when I don't have a free minute? Right? Oh so wrong! They got super weak and the result was a case of bicep tendonitis—a fancy word for lots of pain in my arms that required hours of physical therapy.

MOTIVATION FROM TEAM MALLETT

My arms are amazing now. Since the weather has turned warm,
I'm wearing short sleeves, and the other day my arm caught my eye.
It looked like I was flexing my bicep when in fact my arm was relaxed.
I've never had such toned, nicely shaped arms.
—Robin Wood, 48, Fayetteville, North Carolina

Now, I know you're fired up to work your arms, so I'll wrap this up with just one more reason to tone up top. Build a stronger upper body and you'll stand taller, improve your posture, and enter a room looking more confident. Just think about any woman you know who walks into a room and is commanding, even without saying a word. Guess what all these women have in common? Great body language—and all that starts with great posture. When you *look* more confident, people respond to you very differently. And when that happens, you *feel* more confident. All that from picking up some dumbbells and doing a few minutes of upper-body work each day. Go figure!

QUICK UPPER-BODY BLAST

ABOUT THE WORKOUT

What It Is: This first group of exercises will not only tone your upper body but also work your legs. That's because you have to stabilize your abs and lower body during most of these moves. (Hey, when you're short on time, it's important to get more bang for your exercise buck!) I've also thrown in some ab moves to give the arms a break and whittle down your middle.

How to Do It: Perform 10–15 reps starting with the first exercise, and then proceed to the next exercise. After doing all three exercises once, repeat for a total of three circuits.

It Will Take You: Six minutes per Quick Blast

You Need: 3-pound or 5-pound dumbbells and a fit ball. Increase the amount of weight as you get stronger (for example, as you progress, increase to 5-pound and 8-pound dumbbells). Rule of thumb: If you can easily perform 15 reps, you probably need heavier weights. The last 3 reps should be challenging.

QUICK UPPER-BODY BLAST A

1. Bridge Fly

Inspiration: To give your bust a lift. You won't turn into Dolly Parton (sorry!), but it will help perk up your chest.

Muscles worked: Chest, biceps, glutes, and hamstrings

Reps: 10–15

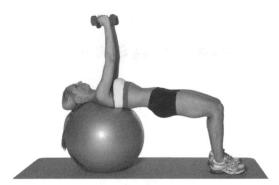 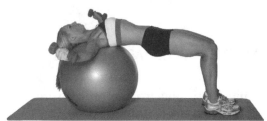

A. Place your shoulder blades and head on the ball. Your legs should be hip-width apart with knees bent. (That is, your body is in a table-top position with your torso in line with your knees.) Reach your slightly rounded arms in front of your chest with the palms facing each other.

B. Inhale and lower arms to shoulder-height, leading with the elbows and without arching the back. Exhale and bring your hands back together, focusing on the chest muscles.

Caution: Lowering your arms past the shoulders places stress on the shoulder joint.

Modification: Perform the exercise without the ball. Instead, lie on your back on the floor with your knees bent and heels level with your sit bones. The spine should be in a neutral position.

Tracey's Tips

• Keep butt muscles and abs contracted and hips in line with knees at *all* times.
• Work toward bringing your legs closer together, which challenges your balance, forcing the abs and hamstrings to work harder to stabilize.

2. Bridge Tricep Extension

Inspiration: Ward off the turkey wobble fat (a.k.a. bat wings).

Muscles worked: Triceps, abs, glutes, and hamstrings

Reps: 10–15

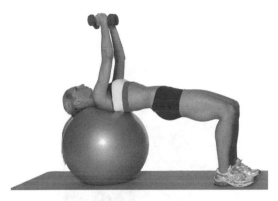 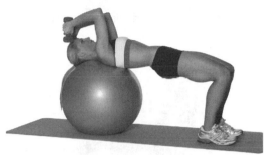

A. Place your shoulder blades and head on the ball with your legs hip-width apart and knees bent (just like in the Bridge Fly). Extend your arms in front of your chest, palms facing each other.

B. Inhale and bend your elbows toward your ears. (Be careful not to hit your face!) Exhale and extend arms back toward the ceiling.

Modification: Perform exercise without the ball. Lie on your back with your knees hip-width apart and your spine in a neutral position.

Tracey's Tips

- Your elbows should be stacked directly over your shoulder joints.
- Move only your forearm and keep the upper arm as still as possible.
- As you fully extend the arms, gently squeeze the triceps for an extra burn.

Active Rest. Place your weights on the floor and perform the following.

3. Abdominal Roll with Reach

Inspiration: The ability to wear low-rise jeans. (Even if you don't want to, knowing you can is a fabulous feeling!)

Muscles worked: Abs, especially the obliques

Reps: 10 on each side, alternating sides

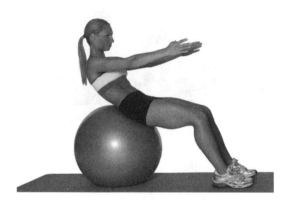 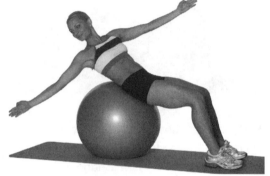

A. Sit on the ball in a deep c-curve of the spine with the small of your back on the ball. Place your feet hip-width apart, knees bent, and arms in front of your body at shoulder height.

Modification: Perform exercise without the ball, sitting tall on the mat with knees slightly bent, hip-width apart.

B. Inhale and twist your torso to the right as you reach your right hand toward the floor, letting your gaze follow it. Exhale and rotate your body back to face forward, maintaining a deep c-curve in the spine. Repeat on the other side.

Tracey's Tip

Keep your hips still as your body rotates. Imagine someone is pulling your right hand, but your left hip is bolted to the ball.

MOTIVATION FROM TEAM MALLETT

My arms got so toned that after just a month,
I had three people say they were amazed at my muscle definition!
—Emily Cole, 28, Euless, Texas

QUICK UPPER-BODY BLAST B

1. Row on the Ball

Inspiration: A sexy back for swimsuits, gowns, and tanks and, oh yeah, better posture!

Muscles worked: Posterior deltoids, rhomboids, lats, and abs

Reps: 10–15

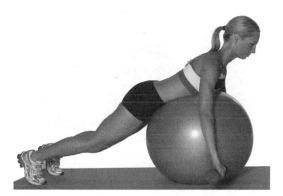
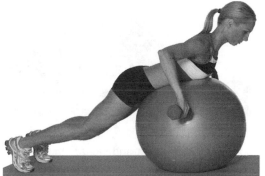

A. Lie face down with your chest resting on the ball, legs extended behind you, knees slightly bent, and toes curled under. Your elbows should be bent to the side of your body in line with your shoulders, and your palms should be facing away from the body.

B. Exhale, lead with your elbows to shoulder height, and squeeze your shoulder blades together. Inhale and lower arms back to the starting position.

Tracey's Tips

• Focus on having the mid-upper back do all the work.

• You shouldn't feel any tension in the head, neck, and shoulders.

• Thanks to upper back muscles that are often weak and stretched out from poor, slumped-over-a-desk posture, it may be hard to do this with weights at first. If so, start with no weights and add them as you get stronger.

2. Preacher Curls

Inspiration: To easily carry your groceries, kids, or those shopping bags brimming with new clothes for your sexy, slim figure!

Muscles worked: Biceps and abs

Reps: 10–15

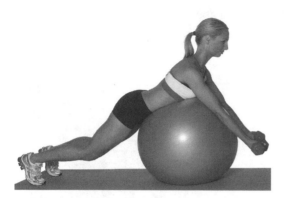 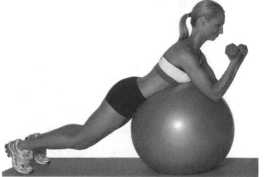

A. Lie with your chest and triceps on the ball, with your arms fully extended and your palms facing upward. Extend your legs behind you, with knees slightly bent and toes curled under, resting on the balls of your feet.

B. Exhale and bend your elbows toward your body. Inhale and fully extend the arms toward the floor.

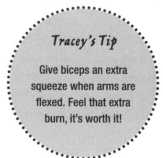

Tracey's Tip

Give biceps an extra squeeze when arms are flexed. Feel that extra burn, it's worth it!

MOTIVATION FROM TEAM MALLETT

I'd been doing the program for just three weeks when I got out of the shower and heard my husband exclaim, 'Wow! I can really see a change in your body!' What could be better than that?
—Leanne Scarcella, 29, Northeastern, Massachusetts

Active Rest. Place your weights on the floor and perform the following.

3. Rabbit on the Ball

Inspiration: Swap your jelly belly for some six-pack abs!

Muscles targeted: Abs and upper body

Reps: 10–15

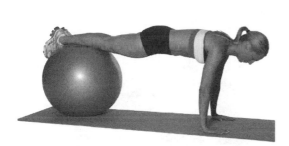

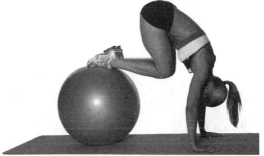

A. Place hands shoulder-width apart on the floor, with legs extended behind the body and shins resting on the ball in a plank position.

B. Exhale, contract your abdominals, and bring your knees toward your chest as you curl your spine like an angry cat. Inhale and extend your legs back out to the plank position.

Modification: Place the ball under the hips for further support. As you gain more strength and confidence, you can move the ball toward the shins.

Tracey's Tips

• Imagine you're drawing your pubic bone toward your belly button and scooping out the abs.
• Be careful not to sink in between the shoulder blades because this may place strain on the shoulder joints. Push away from the floor and pull your shoulder blades down, contracting the lats to stabilize the upper body.

QUICK UPPER-BODY BLAST C

1. Single-Arm Chest Press

Inspiration: Strong upper body; picking up heavy boxes will be a breeze!

Muscles worked: Chest, triceps, hamstrings, glutes, and abs

Reps: 10 on each side, alternating sides

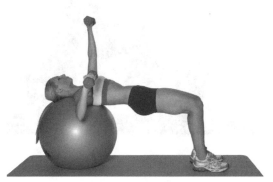

A. Place your shoulder blades and head on the ball, with your legs bent and hip-width apart. (That is, your body should be in a table-top position.) Contract your glutes, making sure that your torso is in line with your knees. Bend your arms so they're perpendicular to the floor, with your elbows in line with your shoulders.

Modification: Perform exercise without the ball with legs bent and hip-width apart and your spine in a neutral position.

B. Exhale and extend your right arm across your chest toward the left side. Inhale and lower the arm back to the starting position. Repeat with the left arm.

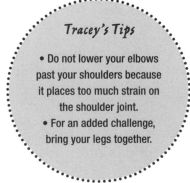

Tracey's Tips

• Do not lower your elbows past your shoulders because it places too much strain on the shoulder joint.

• For an added challenge, bring your legs together.

2. Lateral Raises

Inspiration: Shapely shoulders, which give the illusion of a smaller waist!

Muscles targeted: Shoulders

Reps: 10–15

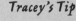

Tracey's Tip

Keep your arms rounded and in your peripheral view. Don't lift them higher than your shoulder joints.

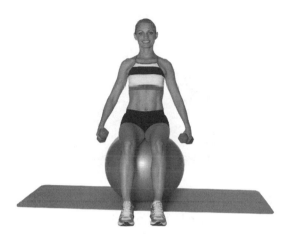 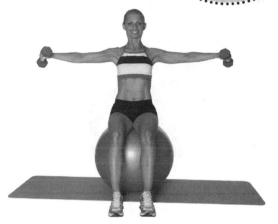

A. Sit tall on the ball with your arms by the sides of your body and feet hip-width apart.

B. Exhale and lift your arms, leading with the elbows, to the sides of your body at shoulder height.

MOTIVATION FROM TEAM MALLETT

I love feeling my shoulders and my arms while I am driving around in the car. I can't believe how much stronger they have gotten! My husband is tired of me asking him to feel them all the time. Plus, I did twelve push-ups on my toes the other day with good form, no sagging bottom!
—Jennifer Thibault, 33, San Marino, California

Active Rest. Place your weights on the floor and perform the following.

3. Side-Overs

Inspiration: To lose the muffin top!

Muscles worked: Obliques

Reps: 8–10 on each side

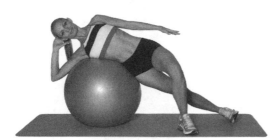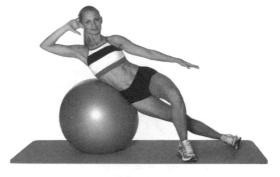

A. Lie on the ball on the right side of your waist and extend your right leg out to the side, with your left leg bent and crossed over the right. Make sure that your left foot is firmly pressed into the floor for support. Place your right hand behind your head and your left arm by your side.

B. Exhale and side bend toward your legs (imagine you're lifting up and over), contracting the sides of your abs to pull yourself up. Inhale and lower back to the starting position.

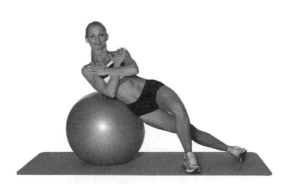

Tracey's Tips

• Don't use your legs or move your hips when lifting your torso to the side. Imagine you're folding the side of your waist.
• Keep your hips facing forwards and stacked on top of each other.

Modification: Cross your arms over your chest, with your hands resting on your shoulders. This will make the exercise easier because it reduces the weight that the body has to curl up.

QUICK UPPER-BODY BLAST D

1. Negative Push-Ups

Inspiration: To finally wear a strapless top! (I call them boob tubes.)

Muscles worked: Chest, shoulders, biceps, triceps, and abs

Reps: 10

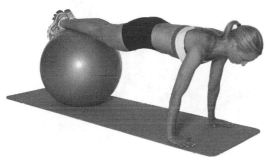 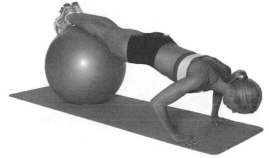

A. Place hands shoulder-width apart with legs extended behind you in a plank position. Shins should be resting on the ball and abs should be contracted.

B. Inhale as you slowly descend toward the floor in a slow count of four, then push up on a count of two. Imagine you're pushing away from the floor and drawing your shoulder blades down your back at the same time. Bend the elbows only as far as you can and still maintain good form (no sinking in between the shoulder blades).

Modification: Perform the exercise without the ball, in a classic push-up position.

Tracey's Tips

• The further the ball is away from your torso—for example, if your shins are on the ball instead of your hips—the more your abs will have to work to stabilize the body.
• Draw your abs in at all times and watch that your lower back doesn't arch.

2. Lat Pull

Inspiration: Being able to wear a backless gown or just a t-shirt without a cami underneath!

Muscles worked: Lats, triceps, and abs

Reps: 10–15

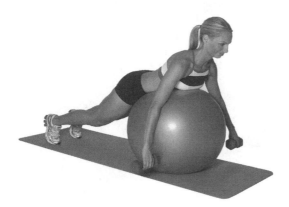 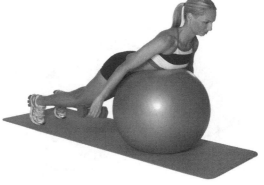

A. Place your chest on the ball, with your legs extended behind you and slightly bent. Curl your toes underneath, resting on the balls of the feet. Place your arms on either side of the ball with your palms facing behind you.

B. Exhale and lift your arms about 6–8 inches toward the hips, keeping the torso completely still. Inhale and return the arms back to the start position.

Active Rest. Place your weights on the floor and perform the following exercise on page 77.

Tracey's Tips

• Try not to use momentum and go slowly through the full range of motion.
• Engage the lats (the sides of the back) by reaching your hands down to the floor and then lifting your arms. This also decreases tension in the neck.

3. Forearm Elbow Balance

Inspiration: A flat, pooch-free belly!

Muscles worked: Abs, glutes, and hamstrings

Reps: 5 each leg

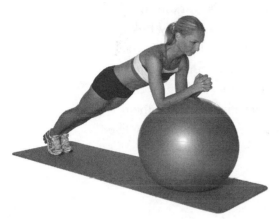

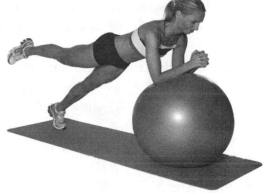

A. Place your forearms on the ball with your hands clasped together. Your elbows should be directly under your shoulders. Extend your legs behind your body with your inner thighs together and your toes curled under.

B. Exhale, contract your abs, and lift your right leg off the floor; then lower it.

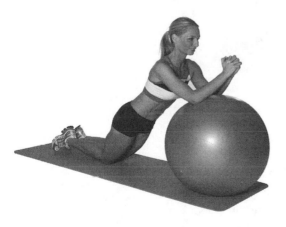

Modification: Hold the plank without moving the legs or kneel on the floor and slightly move the ball forward with your forearms. Instead of doing reps, hold in the modified position for 20–30 seconds.

SHORT AND SWEET STRETCHES

I know you have a million things to do and you've already taken time to work out. But please spend a few minutes stretching your body and cooling down. You may think stretches aren't important, but they're a must for releasing tension in those poor muscles that have worked so hard! Plus, if your muscles are loose and flexible, tomorrow's workout will be that much easier and enjoyable. That's not the only reason why I like to stretch. There are mental benefits, too. I like to think of stretching as a time to collect my thoughts and gear up for the rest of my day. It's the one time I'm actually sitting still and it feels good. Try it. I promise that it helps. Even type A personalities—and I consider myself one of them—need a few moments of serenity. Hold each stretch for thirty to forty-five seconds while taking deep breaths.

Back Stretch

Purpose: To extend and stretch the spine and open the chest

Duration: 30–45 seconds

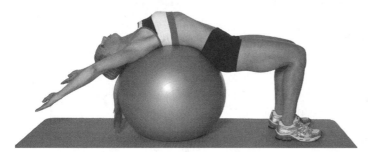

A. Lie face up on the ball with your legs on the floor and your knees bent shoulder-width apart. Extend your arms overhead and toward the floor. Your eyes should be focused toward the back of the room.

B. Slowly roll your body back on the ball as far as is comfortable without straining your neck. For a harder stretch, extend your legs completely. Hold this stretch for 30–45 seconds, and then slowly lower your hips to the floor and carefully roll up through the spine until you are sitting on the floor (off the ball).

Threading the Needle

Purpose: To stretch the lats, obliques, mid back, and lower back

Duration: 30–45 seconds

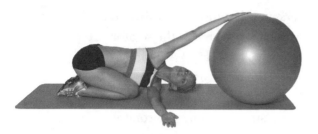

A. Kneel on the floor with both hands on top of the ball, spine extended, and head looking toward the floor.

B. Thread your left arm underneath the right, rotating your torso toward the right side under the arm. Go as far as you comfortably can, and then rest the back of the left shoulder on the floor with your palm facing upward. Hold this stretch before repeating on the other side.

Child's Pose

Purpose: To stretch the back and open the chest and shoulders

Duration: 30–45 seconds

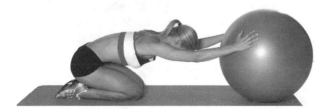

A. Kneel on the floor with both hands on top of the ball and your spine extended. Keep your head in line with your spine and your eyes focused toward the floor.

B. Press your hips back toward your thighs, lengthening and elongating your spine. Gently breathe into the back of the ribcage (this helps open the upper back) as you hold the stretch.

A WEIGHT ON YOUR SHOULDERS

One of the most common upper-body injuries is impingement of the shoulder joint. Boy is it painful. The symptoms are pain in the shoulders and biceps.

What's the cause? Well, your shoulders are big muscles, and when they get strong, they like to take over for weaker ones such as the rotator cuffs (little muscles in the shoulder joint that keep it in place). When that happens, the rotator cuffs get inflamed and the result is pain in your shoulders and biceps.

You can prevent this type of problem by strengthening the rotator cuff muscles, lats, and mid-to-upper back muscles. You should also stretch your chest muscles; this keeps the shoulders from rolling forward and going out of alignment, which also puts strain on the rotator cuffs.

Do the following simple exercise every time you do your arm exercises—at least twice a week.

Rotator Cuff Strengthener

(external rotation)

Reps: Three sets of 10, alternating each side

What You Need: 2-pound or 3-pound dumbbell

Tracey's Tip

• Imagine your shoulder is like a door hinge as you lift your forearm.

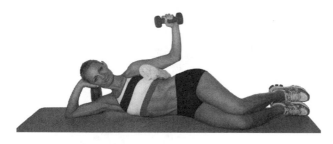

A. Lie on the right side of your body with your knees bent and your bottom arm bent and supporting your head. Place a rolled-up towel between your ribcage and the top (left) arm, and bend your elbow with your palm facing the floor.

B. Exhale and lift your forearm up toward the ceiling, keeping the elbow close to your ribcage. Move only from the shoulder, keeping the elbow at a 90-degree angle. Do a total of 10 reps, switch sides, and repeat.

Chest and Shoulder Stretch

Muscles targeted: Pectorals (chest) and shoulders

Reps: 5

What You Need: Rolled-up towel

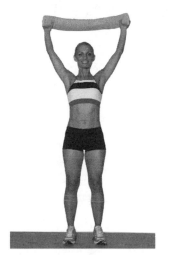

A. Stand tall holding a rolled-up towel in front of your body, with your hands shoulder-width apart.

B. Exhale and lift your arms up and over your head until you feel a stretch in your chest and shoulders. Hold for a few seconds, and then return your arms back to the starting position and repeat.

Tracey's Tip

• Slightly bend your elbows to decrease the pressure on the shoulder joint.

TIPS FROM THE PROS: NO MORE BACK PAIN

Chantal Donnelly, MPT, suggests these tips for preventing back pain:

- **Don't smoke:** People who smoke are 2.7 times more likely to develop low back pain. That's because nicotine causes a thickening of the blood vessel walls, which, in turn, decreases blood flow and oxygen to muscles, bones, and ligaments.
- **Walk with a big stick:** Imagine you have a long pole or stick glued to your back, from your tailbone to the top of your head. Every time you bend over (to brush your teeth, pick something off the floor, and so on), you can hinge only at your waist rather than flexing your spine. This little trick keeps your back in what we call a "neutral spine position" and decreases the everyday wear and tear to your vertebral column.

Success Story

....

Rachel Cronin, 37, Cincinnati, Ohio

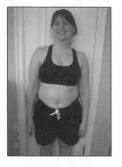 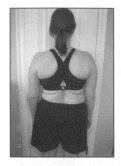 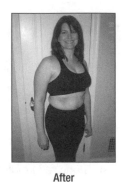 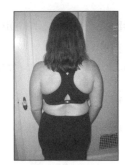

Before   **After**

Lost

13 pounds

Two dress sizes

2 inches off her arms

6 inches off her waist

2 inches off her hips

2 inches off her thighs

12 inches total

Gained

A new motto. *My mantra is, "Why not right now?" when it comes to work-ing out. I had to change my thinking from "I'm too tired to do this" to "I'm too tired not to do this." Inevitably, after twelve minutes, I felt more invigorated, not exhausted! Changing those thoughts has made all the difference.*

• • • • •

Rachel Cronin, 37, had her third baby just two months before starting Tracey's program. She was thrilled about her healthy, new daughter but "felt flabby, squishy, and a little disgusted at the state my body was in," says this high-school English teacher. She had been overweight since childhood—at the age of 12 she had even ordered grapefruit diet pills—

and the extra pounds kept her from feeling confident. Although she had success with exercise and different diets in the past, "I never had any success at actually changing my lifestyle." Part of the problem was her all-or-nothing attitude about exercise. "I thought it wasn't worth it if I didn't have an hour to go to the gym," she says. "And if I *did* have that time, I'd work out so hard that I was too sore to exercise for a week."

After trying Tracey's program, Rachel's attitude—and her body—changed. "I did Tracey's DVD in the morning before work for just twelve minutes. Some days that was all I could fit in, but I learned to embrace the idea that 'something is better than nothing' and it has truly paid off."

Rachel also had to look at some of her eating habits. Fattening snacks such as crackers, cookies, and chocolate were the norm, as were large portions, seconds at dinner, and late-night munching. "Some major changes had to take place, and they were hard at first, but they've become second nature now," she says. One such habit was keeping a food journal. "At first, writing down my food intake was embarrassing, even to myself! Who wants to own up to finishing your child's sandwich? Polishing off a pan of brownies? It was alarming but beneficial," she says. "I learned to plan ahead and be prepared with healthy snacks for myself." She also learned to eat more slowly.

Soon, Rachel realized this wasn't like diets she'd tried before. "In the past, I'd get very gung-ho about something, then drop it a week later," she says. "By the third week, I knew I could stick to Tracey's program because it was easy to fit into my lifestyle." She also learned that eating well takes organization. "It's just too easy to not plan ahead and then grab something sketchy because I'm starving. But when I take fifteen minutes on a Sunday night to chop up veggies and grill chicken breasts for the week ahead, I have a great eating week."

RACHEL'S STICK-WITH-IT TIP

Tell everyone about your plan. I told my husband, kids, parents, and siblings about the program. Just the fact that I told people what I was doing was enough to motivate me to complete the program; the accountability was crucial to my success. Plus, you may tell a friend and find out she wants to join you, too.

Her efforts paid off. When she went back to work after a three-month maternity leave, she easily fit into her pre-pregnancy pants. "My coworkers were shocked (as I was)," says Rachel. "I also got a lot of comments about how I seemed to handle the transition back to work well, and how calm I was for someone still nursing a baby every three hours all night. Losing weight and exercising helped me handle my busy life pretty well. Keeping my moods regulated has been a surprising benefit of the program." Her muscular definition also amazed her. "I found that I actually did have abs hiding under that post-baby tummy," she says. Still, the upper-body workouts were her favorites. "I love the row on the ball because when I first started I couldn't even hold any weights and by the end I was lifting 10 pounds! This was crucial because I needed a stronger upper body to comfortably carry my growing baby.

"When I started the program, I was very skeptical that I could stick with it and that it would even work for me. I'm still amazed that eighteen minutes or so of exercise a day and eating right helped me both physically and mentally," says Rachel. "But I'm a better teacher, friend, wife, and mother now that I've given myself the chance to make these important changes. I'm much more optimistic about my ability to stick with a healthy lifestyle. I feel better at age 37 than I ever did in my 20s. And I look better, too!"

TRACEY'S TAKE

The first picture I saw of Rachel was with her new beautiful baby. They say you can tell a lot about body language, and I noticed that she had conveniently placed her daughter in front of her tummy. I then looked at the next picture, and there she was standing all alone looking not so confident.

Being a new mom and going back to work is an emotional roller coaster. This is usually the time when stress takes over and binge eating starts. Rachel managed to overcome this by combining a small amount of exercise, healthier foods, and the drive to feel sexy again. She proves that something is better than nothing. New moms everywhere, take note!

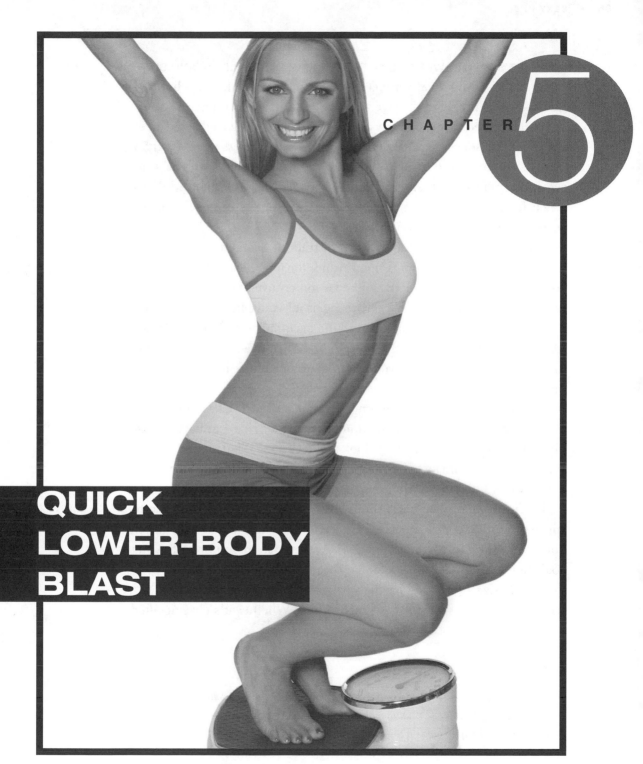

CHAPTER 5

QUICK
LOWER-BODY
BLAST

L ET'S TALK LOWER BODY—THE GOOD OLD HIPS, LEGS, AND BUTT. I don't think I've ever met a woman who said, "I love my butt" or "I love my thighs." Have you? Didn't think so. And that's okay. I admit that I used to feel this way after years of being criticized as a dancer with "athletic soccer legs." Pregnancy didn't help matters when I put 55 pounds on my petite frame. Some days I felt like all that weight went right to my hips, butt, and thighs. As you can imagine, that didn't do much for the old confidence. However, I can honestly say that three years later I truly appreciate my legs.

But what I've realized after years of training women is that loving your butt or hips or thighs is not a reality for most, even if that part of your body does look fabulous. We're far too critical of our body to ever say we love any part of it. Not surprising, is it? We've been programmed from our pre-teen years to emulate all the beautiful and airbrushed photos of women in the media. But I live in Los Angeles and know firsthand that the models and celebs you see in magazines look just like normal people in real life.

Tyra Banks, however, is standing up to the media. She has a beautiful, curvy body! She's proof that you don't have to be a size 4 or have jutting hip bones and sunken cheeks to look and feel sexy. What a relief—especially since the average American woman wears a size 14 (just like Marilyn Monroe did) and half the women in this country are plus-sized.

I believe one of your goals should be to at least like your lower body and feel good in a pair of jeans. You should also know that your lower body will always be a work in progress. And even more importantly, your goal should be to take a big step back from dreaming about fitting your thighs into size 4 jeans and having a perfectly round derriere, and instead appreciate what a strong lower body can do. Whether it's chasing after

MOTIVATION FROM TEAM MALLETT

I have one pair of pants that I've never worn without a body shaper underneath to hold all the jiggly parts in. After just one week on the program, I was shocked that I could put them on without the body shaper! After six weeks, I was loving my ass! I found that I was checking myself out in the mirror every time I walked by.
—Tanya Torforson, 28, Bruderheim, Canada

your kids, running a 5K race, or speed-walking through the mall when there's a sale at your favorite store, it's your lower body that gets you where you want to go.

Why do women dislike their lower bodies so much? One big reason is cellulite, so let's chat about that for a bit. After the birth of my first child and the accompanying weight gain, my legs and butt didn't look so chipper, to put it mildly. One day, I was getting changed after an exercise class in one of those rooms with horrible fluorescent lighting (mistake number one). Even worse, this particular room had mirrors situated all around it. I stepped out of my yoga pants, and there it was in every mirror: a complete profile of my buns. I was in total shock after the first look. After the second, I froze. I couldn't believe that the cottage cheese–ridden skin staring back at me was attached to my body. I know you're all flipping to the front cover, looking at me, and thinking, yeah right! But I couldn't and wouldn't make this up! I don't have a picture of it to convince you (thank heaven!), but let's just say that I totally relate to cellulite.

An estimated 85–95 percent of us have some cellulite; even those skinny-minnies you envy have it. See ladies, we're in this together! The solution would be for all of us to say cellulite is fashionable. It's in! It's hot! That way we'd all feel much better. But until cellulite becomes trendy and makes its way onto the cover of *Vogue* and *Glamour,* we have to do the best we can to make it look better. There is hope, but it's not a jar of cream, a fat-burning pill, or liposuction. (Not only is liposuction extremely painful and expensive, it can actually make cellulite look worse. A lot of pain for not a lot of gain!)

Here's how it happens. Cellulite is caused by fibrous bands that connect the skin to the deeper layer of tissues in the body. These bands

TECHNICAL STUFF: PLYOMETRIC EXERCISES

My Quick Lower-Body Blast contains several plyometric exercises. This fancy word describes exercises that enable a muscle to reach its maximal strength in as short a time as possible. Not to bore you, but the word comes from the Latin words *plyo,* which means increase, and *metric,* which means muscle. (Still awake?) These exercises are great training for sports that require speed-strength, such as tennis, sprinting, soccer, and softball. Wondering why this is important even if you don't play sports and aren't planning to sprint anytime soon? One word: Vanity. Plyometric exercises are another way to challenge the legs and torch calories at the same time. Plus, training your muscles this way helps you function better in daily life whether you have to quickly climb stairs, get out of a chair, or break a fall.

crisscross each other and, as a result, separate the fat that lies beneath them into compartments. A good analogy is a down comforter. Most comforters are stuffed with feathers, which are sewn into puffy, diamond-shaped compartments. The more feathers you have in each compartment, the more it puffs out. When excessive amounts of fat are under the skin, the result is not-so-cute dimples. Unfortunately, as you age and your skin gets thinner and less elastic, the dimples can look even more obvious. The less fat poking through the fibrous bands (the threads on the comforter), the better.

The trick? Losing weight and changing your diet. Not earth-shattering, I know, but that's exactly what I did, and I can honestly say my butt has come a long way. In fact, my friends call me the "Butt Queen." This is my problem spot and I'll always have to work hard to keep it in shape, but I swear the results are worth it! The first step is what this chapter is about: the Quick Leg Blast. These moves will tighten and tone you fast. We'll get to that shortly, but first I want to share a few easy tips to help you find peace south of the border.

The first: Don't try bathing suits on at the store. Those dressing rooms with their horrible florescent lights are enough to give any woman a panic attack. Instead, be kind to yourself and grab a few suits to try on in the comfort of your home, with pleasant lights (that you can dim if you want to), and on your own time rather than in a rushed state you often have in the dressing room. Most stores have flexible return policies, but check to make sure (or order suits online). And then, if you don't like the suits, you can take them back.

The second: A fake tan. Not only is it safer than the sun's dangerous UV rays (which lead to deadly skin cancer, so don't even think about laying out in the sun or on a tanning bed), but it gives you great color in no time flat and your legs will look hot. Plus, it hides cellulite pretty well. I

MOTIVATION FROM TEAM MALLETT

While my husband is always complimentary about my appearance, he has been absolutely obsessed with my new shapely butt. I can be bending over to put clothes in the dryer and he'll be marveling at my new butt. I must admit, it is fabulous!
—Robin Wood, 48, Fayetteville, North Carolina

TIPS FROM THE PROS: PERFECT YOUR FAUX GLOW!

Get a flawless, natural looking fake tan with these tips from Anne Marie Cilmi, director of training at Bliss Spa.

"One of the biggest mistakes people make is using too much tanner," says Cilmi. "It's like seasoning chili. You can always add more, but you can't take out the spice once it's in."

- Exfoliate skin in the shower with a body scrub or loofah. This preps the skin by getting rid of dry flakes so that the self-tanner goes on evenly, looks more natural, and lasts longer. (Avoid oil-based scrubs because their residue prevents the tanner from absorbing.)
- Moisturize only your ankles, heels, kneecaps, and elbows; these areas tend to soak up more self-tanner than the rest of the body and look too dark. The moisturizer prevents excess absorption.
- Wear snug, disposable gloves (available at most drug stores) to avoid orange palms and wrists—a big fake-tan faux pas.
- After putting tanner in your hands, rub palms together so that the tanner spreads evenly.
- Apply tanner using long, full strokes. When the product begins to penetrate, blend it in circular motions.
- Start with your lower body and move up. First, apply tanner to the area between your ankles and knees, and then rub whatever tanner is left on your hands onto your feet, ankles, and knees. These areas have thick skin so they don't need as much tanner to look dark. Next, apply tanner to your thighs and then your stomach. Keep working up the body.
- Wait eight hours after application to apply moisturizer, to shower, or to exercise.

---

swear I felt like I won the lottery the day I discovered that. You can either give yourself a faux glow at home (see tips on this in the "Perfect Your Faux Glow" sidebar) or go to a spa or salon that has a spray tan booth, where a pro spritzes your whole body with self-tanner.

It's truly amazing what an instant tan does for your confidence. It's safe, easy, and you'll love the compliments you get. It's a great way to get bathing-suit-ready for vacation, look your best for a big event (think high school reunion or a hot date), or just like what you see in the mirror every day. I promise you that between the Quick Leg Blast and a fake tan, cellulite will be an almost-distant memory! In fact, at some point, you'll catch a glimpse of yourself in the mirror and think, "I look good."

So let's talk about working out your lower body. I know from my female clients that many women worry that strength training their legs will bulk them up like sausages. This is a general concern women have about weight lifting that I talked about in the preceding chapter, but it bears repeating. Women just don't have the testosterone to bulk up. You may actually weigh more if your legs are muscular versus flabby, but the good news is that muscle takes up less space than fat. That means that the scale may be the same or higher, but your pants will be looser. You may even wear a smaller dress size.

At the beginning of any kind of resistance training program, there may be a slight weight gain from muscle mass. But eventually that extra muscle actually helps your body lose weight because muscles burn more calories than fat (even when your butt is planted firmly on the couch).

The lower body has the largest muscle groups in the body, so you have to work those muscles hard to get results—as well as do cardio to shed fat all over. Let's get started, shall we?

WHO KNEW?

Knees get injured more often than any other joint in the body. And women injure one of the major ligaments in the leg—the anterior cruciate ligament (ACL)—twice as often as men thanks to a combo of hormones and our wider pelvis. Strengthening the hamstrings and muscles around the knee joints and hips helps prevent ACL injuries.

QUICK LOWER-BODY BLAST

ABOUT THE WORKOUT

What It Is: A lower-body circuit that consists of strength exercises and fat-blasting, calorie-burning intervals. There are three Quick Lower-Body Blast workout segments: A, B, and C. You can do one for a six-minute workout, or two for a twelve-minute session, or all three for eighteen minutes.

How to Do It: Do each exercise once before going to the next exercise. Then perform all exercises three times through. If you choose to do more than one Quick Lower-Body Blast workout segment, do a thirty-second march in place between them. (After you get more advanced, you may want to take out the thirty-second march.)

It Will Take You: Six minutes per Quick Blast

Warm-Up: Two to three minutes: March in place or, if you have a staircase, walk up and down the stairs moving your arms in opposition.

QUICK LOWER-BODY BLAST A

1. Traveling Side Squats on Toes

Inspiration: Sexy looking calves and thighs when you wear stilettos.

Muscles targeted: Glutes, hamstrings, quads, and calves

Reps: 8 to the right and left

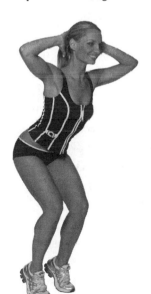

A. Stand on your tip-toes with feet shoulder-width apart. Slightly pitch your torso forward from the hips and bend your knees directly over your first and second toes, so you're in a squat position. Place your hands behind your head.

B. Step out to the side, keeping both knees bent and your body pitched forward. Step two steps to the right and then two steps to the left for one minute.

2. Kick Squats

Inspiration: A butt-i-ful butt that looks perfect in your jeans. Okay, my sense of humor is a bit lame, but I bet you laughed.

Muscles targeted: Glutes, hamstrings, quads, and abs

Reps: 10 front kicks and 10 back kicks, alternating legs

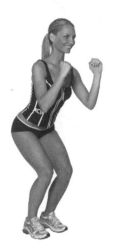 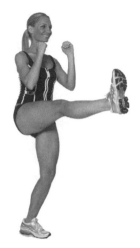 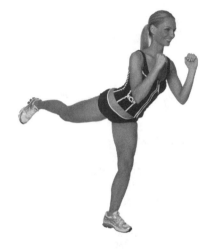

A. Stand with legs shoulder-width apart and knees bent in a squat position, making sure that your body weight is in your heels and your upper body is slightly hinged forward from the hips. Bend your elbows so that your hands are by your face in a boxer's guard position.

B. Exhale as you contract your abs and extend the legs out of the squat (though your legs stay slightly bent). Kick your right leg forward to hip height, flexing the foot. Lower your leg and bend both knees into a squat position. Repeat with the left foot, alternating each leg for a total of 10 reps.

C. Next, repeat the same exercise but this time kick behind the body, alternating each leg for a total of 10 reps. Draw the abs toward the spine to prevent overarching in the lower back when you kick behind.

Tracey's Tips

• Keep your gaze forward. Choose an object in front of you at eye level to focus on throughout. This will help you stay centered and balanced.

• Kick out with the heel and focus on the back of the upper leg.

• Kick your leg only as far as you feel comfortable and can hold your balance.

3. Thirty-Second Interval: Jump Squat Twist

Inspiration: Strong but lean thighs. Find your inner athlete! (Yes, you have one!)

Muscles targeted: Glutes, hamstrings, quads, calves, and obliques

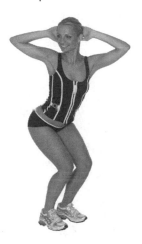

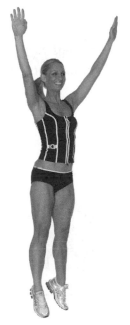

A. Stand with feet shoulder-width apart and knees bent over your first and second toes in a squat position. The weight of your body should be in your heels. Bend your elbows and place both hands behind your head. Twist your torso to the right and left.

B. Reach your hands over your head and propel your body as high as you can off the floor as you extend your legs and jump toward the sky. Land gently through the feet (toe first, then heel) and bend your knees, returning to a squat position with your hands behind your head. Repeat the torso twist right and left.

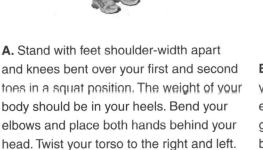

Modification: If you have any knee and back problems, skip the jump and just rise onto your toes without leaving the floor.

Tracey's Tips

• Make it easier on yourself and breathe as you jump.
• Keep your hips facing forward at all times.
• Land through the feet, with your toe first and then your heel. This will help save your joints!
• Land with knees and hips slightly bent. Make sure your knees line up with your toes.

QUICK LOWER-BODY BLAST B

1. Ballet Lunges

Inspiration: Dancer's legs. Need I say more? This is a secret move that I learned from all my years as a dancer, and it really works!

Muscles targeted: Glutes, quads, hamstrings, and inner thighs

Reps: 10 each leg

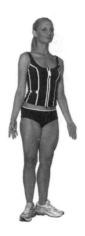

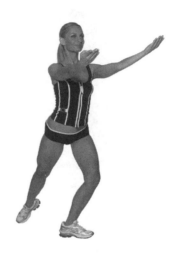

A. Stand tall with your legs turned out at the hips and feet in a small V (like ballet's first position). Place your hands by the side of your body, with your palms facing forward.

B. Inhale and bend your right knee, keeping it in line over the first and second toe. Keep your spine tall as you extend the left leg on the floor behind your body, balancing on a toe. At the same time, reach the arms straight forward to shoulder-height with palms facing upward. Exhale and drag your toe back to the small V position and stand tall.

Tracey's Tip

As you extend the leg behind the body, contract your abs by thinking about zipping up a zipper from your pubic bone to your belly button. This will stop you from arching and placing unnecessary strain on the lower back, and, amazingly, keep you balanced!

Modification: If balance is an issue, hold onto a chair for support.

2. Side Kicks

Inspiration: No more saddlebags! Now you know why I do this move in a lot of my DVDs. The secret's out!

Muscles targeted: Glutes, hamstrings, quads, and abs for stabilization

Reps: 10 each leg

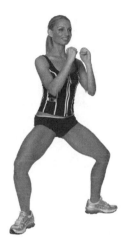
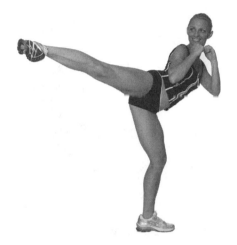

A. Stand with your legs shoulder-width apart in a plié position (your foot are turned slightly outward and your knees are bent). Your knees should be in line with your first two toes and your back should be straight. Bend your elbows, with your fists near your face (as if they're protecting it) in a boxer's stance.

B. Extend your knees and drag your right leg to meet your left leg as you twist your torso slightly to the right. Internally rotate your left leg (the knee is pointing forward) as you lift your knee up until your thigh is parallel to the floor. Kick your left leg out to the left side at hip height. Bring your leg back to the floor and return to a plié position.

Caution: Perform this exercise at a nice even pace, not too fast. It should be a controlled kick, not a ballistic one.

Tracey's Tips

- Imagine you're kicking a door shut with the heel of the foot.
- Keep your knee and shin parallel to the floor.
- Keep your hips and toes facing the opposite direction as you kick to the side. For example, if you kick to the right, your hips and toes face to the left.

3. Thirty-Second Interval: Speed Skate Side to Side

Inspirations: Slipping into a bathing suit and actually liking what you see.

Muscles targeted: Glutes, hamstrings, quads, calves, and obliques

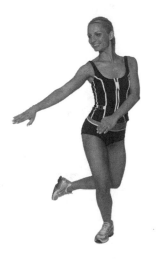

Tracey's Tips

• Keep your knees bent and your body at the same height as you spring side to side.
• Make large steps as you move side to side, forcing the legs to work harder.

A. Stand with your feet shoulder-width apart, knees slightly bent, torso pitched slightly forward from the hips, and your arms by the sides of your body.

B. Step and spring onto your right leg, pushing off your left leg and swinging your arms toward the right side of the body. Repeat, alternating sides, for thirty seconds.

Modification: Don't spring; keep both feet on the floor if you're experiencing discomfort in any joints.

MOTIVATION FROM TEAM MALLETT

Yesterday I tried on a bathing suit that always felt small on me—especially in the behind. I was amazed that it actually fit well around my booty after only three weeks on the program. I'm keeping my fingers crossed that in another three, I'll go from feeling pretty good to fabulous.
—Christine Alfano, 32, Columbia, Maryland

QUICK LOWER-BODY BLAST C

1. Lunge into Warrior One

Inspiration: Beautiful, sculpted thighs!

Reps: 8 each leg

Muscles targeted: Glutes, quads, hamstrings, and abs

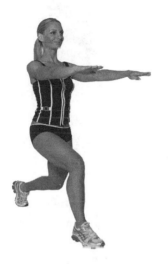

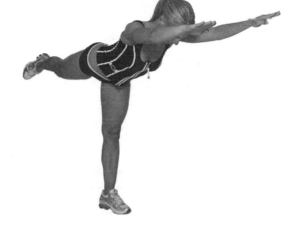

A. Step forward with your right leg into a lunge, with both knees bent and your front knee in line with your toes. Reach both arms forward to shoulder height, palms facing downward.

B. Step back onto your left foot, swing and extend your right leg off the floor behind the body to hip height. The hips, knee, and toes are facing the floor. At the same time, pitch your upper body forward in line with the leg (the T position), with your arms reaching forward overhead in line with your ears.

Modification: Hold onto a chair for support. Or don't elevate the working leg; drag the toe along the floor

Tracey's Tip

Keep your hips level and your abs contracted throughout the exercise to help your balance.

2. Plié Pulses

Inspiration: Perky bottom, as they say in England!

Muscles targeted: Quads, hamstrings, glutes, and abs

Reps: Two sets of 10 pulses in each position

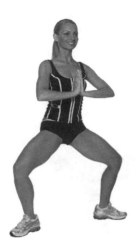 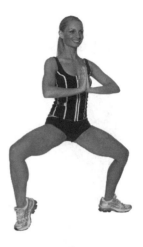

A. Stand with your legs shoulder-width apart, turned out at the hips. Point your feet toward the corners of the room and bend your knees. Bend your elbows, pointing outward, and press the palms together in front of your chest. Hold this position and make little pulses (tiny up and down movements).

B. Lift your right heel off the floor and pulse for 10. Lower your right heel down to the floor. Repeat, lifting your left heel off the floor. Continue one more set, right then left.

Modification: Limit the range of motion.

Tracey's Tips

- Only perform small pulses to keep the work in the thighs.
- Draw abs in toward the spine and don't arch the lower spine. Think of a neutral spine.

MOTIVATION FROM TEAM MALLETT

My daughter was sick and home from school so I couldn't go to the gym or go running. Instead, I did the whole Quick Lower-Body Blast. I was drenched in sweat and amazed at the great workout I had! I also provided entertainment for my daughter because she loved watching me exercise.
—*Wendy Pratt, 38, San Marino, California*

3. Thirty-Second Interval: Running Plank

Inspiration: Total body tune-up in thirty seconds!

Muscles targeted: Quads, glutes, hip flexors, hamstrings, abs, and upper body for support

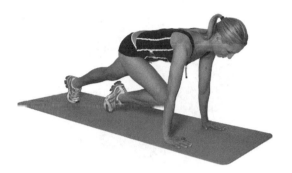

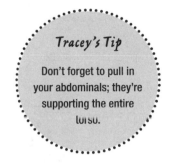

Tracey's Tip

Don't forget to pull in your abdominals; they're supporting the entire torso.

A. Place your hands shoulder-width apart, with your shoulders directly over your hands and your body extended in the plank position. Your toes should be curled under, resting on the balls of your feet.

B. Draw your right knee toward your chest and then extend it back as you spring onto the other foot. (It's like running in place with your hands on the floor.) Keep your shoulders over your hands and your upper body still, with your butt no higher than your shoulders.

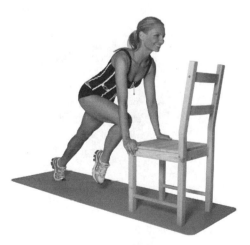

Modification: Elevate your body by holding onto the corner of a chair or a step, and go slower (like walking in place without a spring in your step).

QUICK STRETCHES

1. Hamstring Stretch with Towel

Purpose: Stretch the hamstrings

Hold: 30–45 seconds

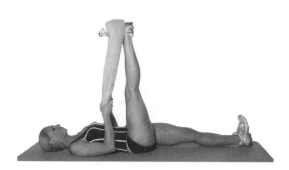

A. Lie on your back with a towel wrapped around your right foot and your left leg extended on the floor. Gently bring your right leg closer to your chest until you can feel the stretch in the back of your leg. Keep your pelvis still in a neutral position while stretching the leg. Switch legs and repeat.

Modification: Bend the supporting leg on the floor if you feel pain in the lower back.

2. Quad Stretch

Purpose: Stretch the front of the thighs

Hold: 30–45 seconds

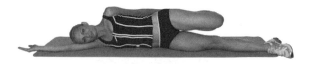

A. Lie on the right side of your hip with the left leg bent. Hold onto the left foot with the left hand and gently pull the leg toward the butt until you feel the stretch in the front of the thigh. To avoid arching the back, draw the abs in toward the spine. Switch legs and repeat on the other leg.

3. Sitting Cross-Leg Stretch

Purpose: Stretch the glutes and open the hips

Hold: 30 seconds

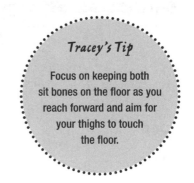

Tracey's Tip

Focus on keeping both sit bones on the floor as you reach forward and aim for your thighs to touch the floor.

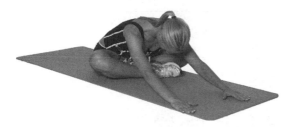

A. Sit tall with your legs turned out at the hips and both knees bent, with your right leg in front of your left leg. Reach your hands in front of your legs on the floor and lift your collarbone up toward the ceiling. Slowly lower your torso until you feel the stretch in the glutes. Hold this position and take deep breaths. Repeat with the other leg in front.

FOUR WAYS TO BOOST YOUR BUTT BURN

1. Contract and release the glutes continuously for two minutes at a time when you're commuting to work, or stand and hold onto a chair and perform side lifts while you're on the phone. Don't feel stupid (though I'd close the door at the office); just visualize your butt in those tight jeans!
2. Always perform glute exercises to fatigue (that is, until you feel like you can't possibly do any more).
3. Do cardio activities that work the butt area, such as hiking, walking a hilly route, biking, or roller skating.
4. Your mind is a powerful tool for maximizing the effectiveness of any exercise, so think about your butt while you're working it. This way, other muscles such as the quads and hamstrings (which are usually stronger) are less likely to take over.

Success Story

•••

Liz Price, 37, married, stay-at-home mother of two,
South Pasadena, California

Lost

15 pounds

4½ percent body fat

Two dress sizes

½ inch off her arms

3 inches off her waist

3 inches off her hips

1½ inches off her legs

8 inches total

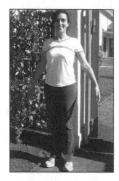
Before

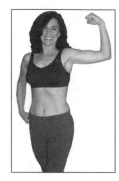
After

Gained

A figure she had never dreamed of. *I truly didn't know that this body was a possibility for me. I thought I was working to maintain where I was, not knowing that I had a slimmer, healthier body inside! I will be doing this program for the rest of my life.*

• • • • •

Liz Price, 37, was one of the few women who didn't join Team Mallett to lose weight. At 5 feet 5 inches, she had always been slim, with a weight that hovered between 126 and 140 pounds for most of her adult life and around 135 pounds in the last few years. In fact, Liz thought she was in pretty good shape. "I was already doing four to five days a week of cardio—the elliptical machine, spinning, or walking—and thought my body was fine. Perhaps a little soft around the midsection, but otherwise I thought it looked pretty good," says this mother of two from South Pasadena, California. She also thought of herself as a healthy eater. "I already ate good foods and definitely thought that exercise was more important than my diet in terms of making changes in my body. I was very hesitant to believe that food would make a big difference for me."

Still, she wanted to build muscles and tone up by adding strength training to her workouts, so she signed on to Tracey's program. "I was also self-conscious about my tummy because I'd always hated my pooch," she says. The changes in her workouts were bigger than Liz expected. "Now my exercising is more efficient. I'm doing fewer cardio workouts, but the ones I'm doing are more effective," she says. "I can't count how many times I've promised myself that I was going to do some sit-ups every day to try to get my stomach flatter. But I've never made it more than a day or two. Tracey's program made it easy to do. In fact, if I skip a day or take my rest on Sundays, I actually miss my ab work!"

Just as surprising was the fact that Liz did need to change her diet. Although she still enjoys the occasional dessert when her family goes out—after all, she doesn't want to feel deprived—she realized that her old so-called healthy eating habits were anything but. "I learned that when you eat is as important as what you eat and that I wasn't eating a balanced diet or getting enough protein to keep my body running efficiently," she says. "Now I think about everything that I eat in terms of how it fits into the larger plan for the day. I used to eat a small amount of ice cream every night for a treat and could eat a whole bread basket, but my cravings for sweets and white flour are totally gone."

The program also taught Liz the importance of mixing up her diet instead of eating the same foods. "Now I vary what I eat for breakfast, incorporating oatmeal, smoothies, or eggs, instead of the cereal I used to eat every single day," she says. "And I eat a lot more protein than before—such as salad with chicken for lunch and dinner." *Sexy in 6* also taught Liz the important art of snacking. "Now I'm never without a morning and afternoon snack. I look forward to them and plan them into

LIZ'S STICK-WITH-IT TIP

Don't pick and choose parts of Tracey's program; do the entire program.
I'd hear some Team Mallett members say, 'I'm not really doing the food plan—
just trying to eat healthier,' or, 'I'm exercising more, but I'm not doing her exercises.'
This misses the point and I wasn't surprised when they didn't get great results.
What you learn through doing Tracey's program is that what you thought was
good eating and exercise isn't really working. Commit to doing her program
her way and you will get results.

my day," she says. "Keeping my blood sugar balanced has resulted in fewer dips in energy midday and a decline in cravings."

Just weeks after starting Tracey's program, Liz said her body started to change shape and the pounds were "dropping off." "By the second week, people were asking me if I'd lost weight," says Liz, who was beyond stunned when she went on her first shopping trip five weeks into the program. "All of my regular clothes were starting to get baggy and look bad, so I tried on one size smaller than normal," she says. "They seemed to fit, but not quite, so I went down another size. I couldn't believe it, but I went from a size 6 to a size 2!" Liz is also amazed at the changes in her lower body. "I always thought I was built a little wider around the hips and that I just had to accept that. But I noticed a huge difference in my butt and hips during this program. I had no idea that they could be so much slimmer!"

With her stomach pooch long gone and a belly that's as flat as it was in her early twenties before having two kids, Liz is no longer self-conscious. "I could actually wear a bikini if I wanted to," she exclaims. Today, Liz has more energy than ever and sleeps more soundly than she has in years. "Most of all, I'm really proud of myself for sticking with this six-week program and proud of my body for how strong it is and what it can do! I feel confident and powerful."

TRACEY'S TAKE

I first met Liz about two years ago at our local YMCA, where she would take my Saturday morning spinning class. I could see her trying really hard, but she never seemed to be getting the results she wanted. She was stuck in a rut and not working out efficiently. Cardio alone for Liz was not going to get her into the bikini she so longed for. When I asked her to join Team Mallett, she jumped with joy. I contribute Liz's success to her will to succeed and giving her all to this plan. I've watched her body completely change and her confidence grow. She is one hot momma!

CHAPTER 6

QUICK
ABS
BLAST

CREDIT MORE THAN TWENTY YEARS OF DANCE CLASSES FOR helping train my tummy. I remember my first ballet teacher, Cynthia Knowles. She was always telling me to pull my abs in, and when I didn't, she'd remind me, gently tapping a bony finger on my belly as I was dancing. In time, sucking in my gut was second nature and all that contracting of my ab muscles toned my midsection.

Who doesn't love the look of strong abs in a bikini or low-rise jeans? But the benefits are more than skin deep. Did you know that your abs are responsible for supporting your spine? This may explain why some of you experience back pain. I guarantee that if more people did a little more ab work (as well as flexibility training with their hamstrings and hip flexors), we'd see a lot fewer back problems—something about 80 percent of people in Western countries experience at some point in their lives. The abs are connected to the back (this entire area is what people are referring to when they talk about the "core"). When the abs aren't strong, neither is the back.

I can explain it a little better with some science talk (don't worry; you don't need to remember high school biology). The main two muscles responsible for supporting the back are the transverse abdominal muscle and the multifidus (say those words ten times fast!). The transverse abdominal muscle is the deepest of four layers of abdominal muscles. The multifidi are very short muscles on the sides of the vertebra (a.k.a. the spine) and running up to the middle of the back. Research from the University of Queensland in Australia shows that those of us without back problems start any movement of our arms or legs with a contraction of the transverse abdominal and the multifidus, a sign that the brain is prepping the back for the stress involved in taking action. This does not happen, however, in people *with* back pain, meaning that these muscles are

MOTIVATION FROM TEAM MALLETT

My core muscles are definitely a lot stronger since starting the program three weeks ago—especially my obliques. I've always been stronger on my right side, but I'm now equally as strong on my left side. It's an amazing feeling when you turn the corner on exercises that previously seemed unachievable.
—Laurie Jardin, 43, Ontario, Canada

not supporting the spine before movement. The result is a boost in stress on the back and, hence, the back pain.

The moral of the story? You have to target the transverse abdominal and multifidus muscles not only to get a flat, fabulous looking stomach but also to help improve the ability of these muscles to support and protect the spine. In the end, this can reduce or even prevent an aching back. Plus, a strong core will make it a whole lot easier to do daily activities, from lifting your kids to tying your shoelaces.

Unfortunately, good-looking six-pack abs do not necessarily translate to strong ones. I can say this from experience. I've always had a flexible back. But as it turns out, I had little of the internal core support essential for warding off injuries. I had lower back pain from an over-flexible back and not using my internal support (core) to carry me through dance moves, especially deep back bends, when I was dancing professionally. My back pain decreased after I learned how important it was to activate my deep core muscles while performing abdominal work.

THE SIMPLE SECRET TO GREAT ABS

I'm going to share a major secret with you. Something few people know about, but absolutely key to flatter abs. It's crucial if you want to say good-bye to a stomach pooch or a hard-to-find waist. The amazing thing about this secret is that it's so simple. *Super* simple. Drum roll please . . . The key to great abs is to pretend you're stopping the flow of urine while peeing. Lovely, I know. That's it! But let me explain.

When doing any ab exercise, you can intensify the abdominal contraction simply by activating your pelvic floor muscles. It makes your ab workout that much more effective (and you are improving your sex life at

MOTIVATION FROM TEAM MALLETT

I actually feel the tightness in my abdominals. It's like I'm tightening them even though I'm not. It's a weird feeling I've never had before, but it's cool. I love being able to bend over or lean to one side without feeling a roll of fat bulge over the side of my pants!
—Robin Wood, 48, Fayetteville, North Carolina

the same time; see chapter 9 for more). As you draw in the abdominals, think of pulling up your deep pelvic muscles at the same time. (I think of the two actions as an elevator zipping up to the top floor.) This is exactly what your pelvic floor muscles do when you're trying to stop the flow of urine while waiting in line for the bathroom. I know, it's not a pretty way to describe it, but it's the clearest. These muscle contractions are called kegels. If you've had children you should be familiar with them; if not, you had better read fast. Doing kegels in combination with ab work targets your deep core muscles and intensifies the contraction (the burn).

Think of the abs and the core like a canister. Your transverse abdominal muscle (the front part of the canister) is pulling toward the spine, the pelvic floor (the bottom) is pulling up, the sacral multifidus (the back) is bracing the spine, and finally the diaphragm (the top) is pulling down. When all these muscles work together, they create a strong stable core and amazing abs. *Now* add some deep breathing along with engaging your core—exhaling when you're in the hard part of a movement (drawing in the abs to the spine) and inhaling on the way out of it. A great exercise to target the multifidus is Cat Cow Leg Extension, on page 151.

If this feels a little overwhelming, just take baby steps. As I tell my clients all the time, "Rome wasn't built in a day." Neither are six-pack abs. Just have patience and you'll get there. It's not a hard task when the reward is a toned tummy or a waist you haven't seen in a while. You won't have to suck in your stomach to zip up your favorite jeans. In fact, you might even give the low-rise variety a chance. The first time I truly engaged my core correctly, my abs were shaking like an earthquake; this was a light bulb moment. The difference it made was huge. I whittled my middle and got stronger obliques. Because the transverse abdominal muscle is attached to the internal and external obliques, in working this

MOTIVATION FROM TEAM MALLETT

I can't believe how quickly your abs strengthen when you do the six-minute circuits every morning. I can really tell a difference, even after two weeks! My tummy is flatter and more defined on the sides. After being pregnant three times, I didn't think it was possible to tone my abs like this!
—Marie Queen, 40, San Marino, California

newfound muscle I was getting more bang for my belly-buffing buck. On a side note, this is also great for strengthening the lax pelvic floor after pregnancy.

Drawing in your abs and pulling up your pelvic front are crucial during any ab workout, but you can also do this exercise throughout the day, when you're stuck in traffic, sitting in a meeting, or waiting in line. Here's how: Inhale through your nose and feel the ribcage expand. Then, as you exhale through the mouth, draw your abdominals in toward the spine and pull your pelvic floor up like an elevator. Imagine that as you wait for your son at soccer practice or sit in the pickup line at school, you're working your way to taut, toned abs. I swear, I've had strong athletes, 6-foot 6-inch football players and many skeptics near tears after performing simple abdominal crunches this way. I love it because it means that you don't need to do hundreds of sit-ups to get sleek, sexy abs. You just need the correct technique (in this chapter) and the motivation (wearing a thong or bikini; enough for you?).

TAKE NOTE AND LOOK WHAT THE RESEARCH IS SAYING

Whittling your middle is also important for better health. A study of 42,000 women conducted at the University of Kentucky Medical Center (part of the well-known Nurses' Health Study) found that women with waistlines measuring 36 inches or more were almost twice as likely to require surgery to remove gallstones (solid masses made of cholesterol that form in your gallbladder) than those whose waists came in at 26 inches or less. Another study by researchers at New York–Presbyterian Hospital/Columbia found that women with waistlines of 35 inches or greater were more likely to have high blood pressure and high total cholesterol, low "good" cholesterol, and elevated blood glucose levels—all risk factors for heart disease. In addition, a strong, slim core is responsible for better sports performance—in other words, beating your husband at tennis or your own time in a 5K—and better balance and posture. Now that's something I'm sure you can stomach!

I'm sure you've heard this before, but it's quality not quantity that counts, which is why the Quick Abs Blasts work so well. You're not wasting time using the incorrect muscles or doing an endless number of reps. I can't tell you how empowering it is for so many of my female clients to find their abs—especially after pregnancy or a life of longing for a flatter stomach. Team Mallett was stunned by this. Many have flatter abs at the age of 30 or 40 than they did in their teens and 20s *before* they had kids! However, it doesn't happen overnight. (Sorry!) It's like building a house. You start by building a strong foundation and the rest follows. Without a strong core, the rest of the body is weak.

First let's go over a few pointers regarding correct technique.

BREATHING 101

Isn't it amazing that we breathe all day long, but most of us don't know how to do it? Typically, we take short breaths and don't even *begin* to tap into our lung capacity. What a shame! Proper breathing sends oxygen throughout the entire body, energizes the mind and body, and cleanses the body of impurities. The beauty of Pilates breathing is that once you understand the concept, it becomes second nature. I have to warn you that at first it will feel foreign, maybe even impossible. You'll feel like you're breathing at the opposite time you're supposed to, kind of like patting your head and rubbing your tummy at the same time. However, if you don't breathe properly, you're not activating the deep abs and therefore not working them as effectively. Take a seat and try this:

Step one: Place your hands around your rib cage and relax your shoulders.

Step two: Inhale through the nose, filling the lungs with air. Expand your rib cage, moving your hands outwards.

Step three: Exhale through the mouth as the lungs deflate, drawing the ribs together. Scoop out the abdominals by drawing them toward the spine, like a seat belt tightening across the midsection.

Can you feel those abs work? You can do this exercise in the car, or waiting in line at an ATM or at the grocery store. The more you do it, the

MOTIVATION FROM TEAM MALLETT

I'm exhausted, but I'm having fun and my abs are tighter already after just two weeks.
—*Leanne Scarcella, 29, Rowley, Massachusetts*

more the ab muscles will cooperate and pull in. With this trick, who needs one of those tummy body shapers?

KEEP YOUR SPINE NEUTRAL

While you're doing any kind of ab work, your spine needs to be in what is called a neutral position—in other words, its natural state. It's important to strengthen the spine the way it is actually used or should be used. For example, when we're doing traditional ab crunches, the spine should have a slight curve just like it does when we're standing up. Contrary to popular belief, pressing the lower back into the floor compresses that area, which can cause injury and unnecessary pain. Still, most of us do this because the bigger muscles such as the glutes tend to take over and force the hips to tilt. Instead, if you keep your pelvis still and focus on using the abs to pull your head and neck off the floor, all the effort will be purely in your abs.

Here's how to get into position.

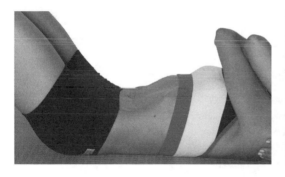

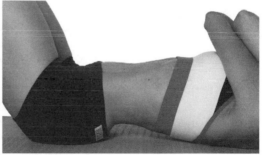

1. Tilt the pelvis: Lie on your back with your knees bent and your heels level with the sit bones (those little bones you, well, sit on). Draw your abs in toward your spine and imagine you're leading with the pubic bone, tilting the pelvis forwards in a tucked (posterior) position.

2. Arch the spine: Arch the spine by arching the pelvis in the opposite direction.

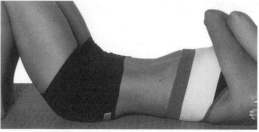

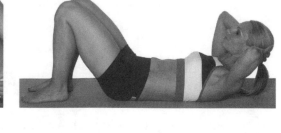

3. Keep a neutral spine: A neutral spine is somewhere in the middle of the two previous positions; just relax the spine and see where it naturally lies. Place your hands on hip bones and pubic bone; you should feel a perfect triangle that's flat to the sky. Imagine you're balancing a cup of water on your tummy. Yes, you will feel a slight arch in the back. Don't worry; this is how your spine is naturally supposed to be; we need curves in our spine for shock absorption.

4. The incorrect form: Here's what happens when you do a classic crunch while tucking the pelvis versus keeping the pelvis in a neutral position.

In this picture, you can see how I'm curling my pelvis under and flattening my spine as I lift my head, neck, and shoulders off the floor. The problem is that I'm overcompensating for weak deep abdominals (transverse abdominals) by letting my glutes and rectus abdominus (the pretty six-pack muscle) do most of the work.

Tracey's Tip

In the correct form, my hips stay still as my head, neck, and shoulders lift off the floor. Now by disengaging the glutes and drawing in my abdominals, all the work is in the abs. Yippee! I can finally feel the burn in my abs.

QUICK ABS BLAST

ABOUT THE WORKOUT

What It Is: Quick Abs Blast A is a fusion of Pilates-based exercises and classic abdominal work. The perfect combo to target the midsection.

Quick Abs Blast B is a series of ab moves performed on an exercise ball. This is a wonderful tool for that extra challenge because the unstable surface forces your deep ab muscles to work so that you can maintain your balance.

How to Do It: Do each exercise once through before going to the next exercise. Remember to engage those pelvic floor muscles by pulling the pelvic floor up and drawing in the abs as you exhale with exertion. The pelvic floor will naturally relax on the inhale as your head goes down.

It Will Take You: Six minutes per segment

You Need: A mat and an exercise ball for Quick Blast B

MOTIVATION FROM TEAM MALLETT

*Last night, my husband was following me up the stairs
and he said that he noticed a difference in my body shape.
This morning, my 7-year-old told me that I looked 'way fitter'
than before! Pretty good for less than a week on the program!*
—Sally Teiniker, 32, Auckland, New Zealand

QUICK ABS BLAST A

1.Circle Roll-Up

Inspiration: Get rid of the Michelin Man–like tire around your belly

Muscles targeted: Abdominals

Reps: 5 each direction

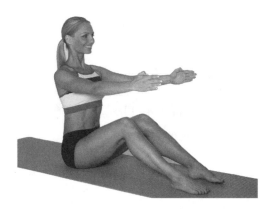
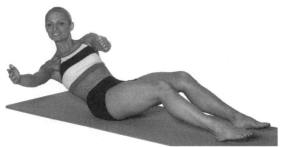

A. Sit tall with your knees bent, your feet hip-width apart, and your spine in a neutral position. Extend your hands forward, in line with your shoulders.

B. Inhale and rotate to the right, moving your arms toward the right side of your body. Roll down the right side of your body through each vertebra until you're lying on your back with your arms overhead.

Exhale and lift your head, neck, and shoulders off the floor, rotating to the left and shifting your hands to the left side of your body. Continue rolling up through the spine, reaching toward your left side and returning to the starting position.

Tracey's Tip

Place a rolled-up towel between your legs. This forces you to activate your inner thighs, which helps target your pelvic floor and abs more effectively.

Modification: Lift only your head, neck, and shoulders off the floor and rotate through your upper body without rolling up through the spine.

2. Dipping the Toes

Inspiration: No more belly fat!

Muscles targeted: Abdominals

Reps: 10 each leg then 5 both legs

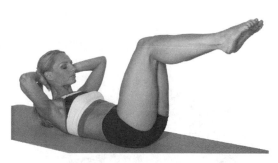

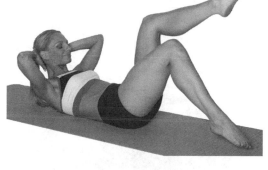

A. Lie on your back with your legs at a 90-degree angle, your shins parallel to the floor, and your knees directly over your hips. Your elbows should be bent, with your hands behind your head. Lift your head, neck, and shoulders off the floor. Focus your eyes toward your belly button, with your chin off your chest.

B. Exhale and contract your abs while dipping your right toes toward the floor. Keep your leg at a 90-degree angle, only moving from your hip joint. Inhale, return your leg back up, and repeat with the other leg. After performing singles, dip *both* legs down.

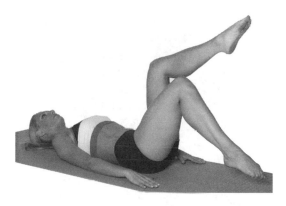

Tracey's Tips

Every time you lower your leg toward the floor, imagine a seat belt tightening over your midsection to keep you from moving your hips and to keep your spine from arching.

Modification: Keep your head on the floor with your arms to the sides of your body.

3. Froggies

Inspiration: Sleek abs and inner thighs. Think shorts!

Muscles targeted: Abs and inner thighs

Reps: 10–15

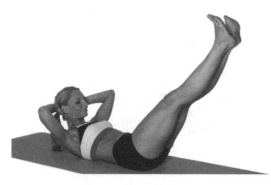

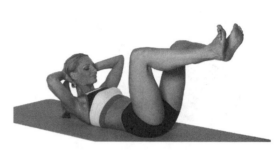

A. Lie on your back with your head, neck, and shoulders off the floor, your hands resting behind your head, and your elbows bent. Turn your legs out at the hips and place your heels together in a small V. Extend your legs diagonally out as far as you can, maintaining good form without arching your lower back.

B. Inhale and bend your knees toward your ears like a frog, without moving the pelvis and upper body. Exhale and extend your legs out, squeezing your inner thighs together.

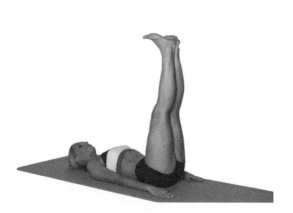

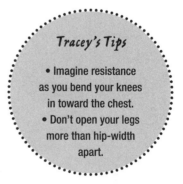

Tracey's Tips

• Imagine resistance as you bend your knees in toward the chest.
• Don't open your legs more than hip-width apart.

Modification: Extend your legs straight up to a 90-degree angle. Keep your head, neck, and shoulders on the floor and your arms by the side of your body.

4. Abdominal Openings

Inspiration: To be able to sit down and not feel a roll of flesh touch the thighs!

Muscles targeted: Abs and inner thighs

Reps: 10

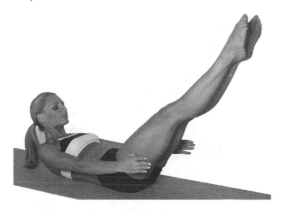

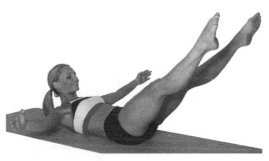

A. Inhale to prepare, and then exhale and lift your head, neck, and shoulders off the floor, reaching your arms out to the sides of your body. Extend your legs out to where you can hold with good form, turning them out at the hips in a small V.

B. Inhale and open your arms and legs out to the sides of your body. Your legs should open to shoulder-width and your arms should be in line with your shoulders. Exhale and contract your abdominals, drawing your arms and legs back together. Repeat 10 times without lowering your head.

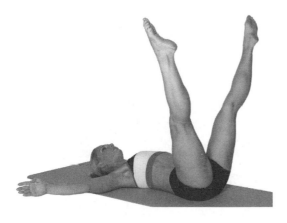

Tracey's Tips

• Imagine drawing an angel in the snow.
• Don't open your legs too wide because this will take the emphasis off your abdominals. Instead, keep the range of motion to shoulder-width apart.

Modification: Extend your legs up to 90 degrees.

5. Side Plank Twist

Inspiration: A shapely waist!

Muscles targeted: Obliques and lats

Reps: 5 each side

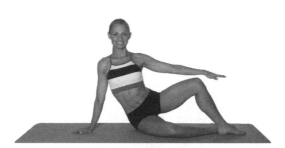

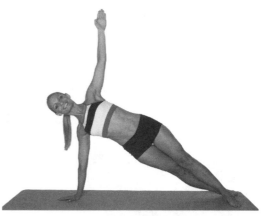

A. Lie on your right hip with your knees bent to the side of your body and your left leg crossed in front of your right leg, with your left foot firmly pressed to the floor. Place your right hand directly under your right shoulder, with your fingers pointed away from your body and your left arm resting on your left hip.

B. Inhale and lift your hips off the floor, extending your legs straight out to the side, with your right arm straight. Lift your left arm straight up toward the ceiling, keeping it in line with your shoulder with the palm facing outward.

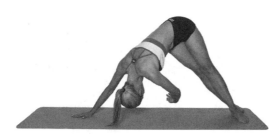

C. Exhale, contract your abs, and twist your upper body toward the floor. Reach your left arm under the supporting right arm, without moving your hips. Inhale and return to the side plank. Bend knees and lower hips toward the floor back to start position and repeat.

Tracey's Tips

• Pull your shoulders away from your ears by focusing on your lats; this also helps you activate the obliques (waist) more efficiently.
• Lower your hips gently with control; it's almost as if the hips skim the floor before going back up into the side plank.

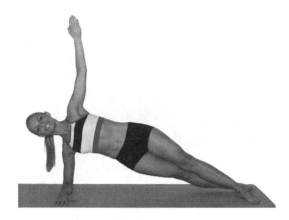

Modification: Balance on your forearm with your fingertips facing forward and your forearm on the floor. Do not rotate your upper body.

6. Plank to Downward Dog

Inspiration: Great set of pins!

Muscles targeted: Abs and hamstrings

Reps: 8–10

Tracey's Tips

• Keep your weight out of your hands by pushing away from the floor, contracting the sides of the back (the lats), and pulling your abs. Your body will feel lighter if it's not pushing dead weight. • Imagine that your abs, not your hip flexors, are drawing your hips into the pike position.

A. Place your hands shoulder-width apart, with your legs extended behind you and your toes curled under in a plank position. Contract your abs and maintain a straight line from the crown of your head to your heels.

Inhale and bend your elbows in a classic push-up, without sinking between the shoulder blades. Exhale and return to the plank position. Inhale and hold the plank for a few seconds.

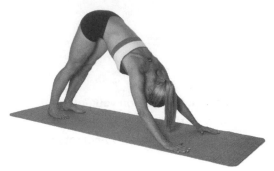

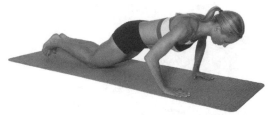

B. Exhale and lift your hips to the sky, extending your spine to a downward dog position and pressing your heels into the floor. Inhale and return to the plank position without moving your hands.

Modifications: You can do the push-up on your knees. Also, it's fine if you're unable to extend your hamstrings in downward dog. Just do as much as your body will allow.

7. Roll-Down

Inspiration: No more lower-back aches and pains!

Purpose: Gentle traction of the spine to release stress in the back

Reps: 1–2 roll-ups, then repeat once

A. From the preceding plank position, walk your hands to your feet and roll up through the spine, contracting the abs and uncurling the head last.

B. Roll down through each vertebra, starting with your chin to your chest, until your hands reach the floor.

C. Let your upper body relax with a slight bend in your knees, and then slowly roll up. This releases stress and tension throughout the spine and leaves you with perfect posture to carry you throughout the day.

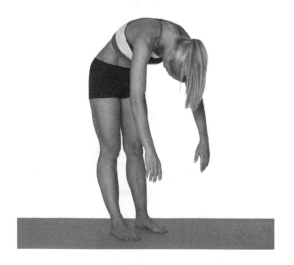

QUICK ABS BLAST B

1. Jab Cross on the Ball

Inspiration: No more roll of fat over your tight pants!

Muscles targeted: Obliques

Reps: 20, alternating sides

A. Lie with the small of your back on the ball and your legs bent, knees hip-width apart. Bend your elbows with your hands in front of your face (boxing stance).

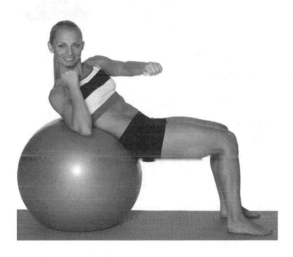

B. Exhale, twist and jab your right arm across to the left side of your body. Keep your eyes focused on your right hand.

Tracey's Tips

• Rotate your upper body by reaching out with the jab.
• Maintain a deep C-curve in the spine throughout the entire exercise. This will keep your abs engaged.

WHO KNEW?

Beat belly bloating by drinking more water. It may sound counterintuitive, but water flushes waste out of your system and keeps things moving if you're constipated (a common cause of a puffy tummy). Other culprits of a bloated stomach are chewing gum and drinking from a straw because they cause you to swallow too much air.

2. Chest Lift with Arm Reach

Inspiration: Washboard abs!

Muscles targeted: Abs

Reps: 10

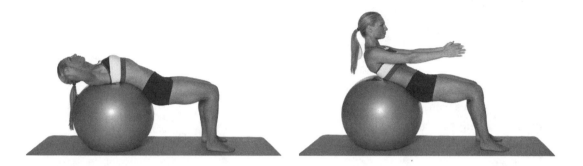

A. Lie with the small of your back on the ball and your legs bent, knees hip-width apart. Bend your elbows and rest your hands behind your head.

B. Exhale and lift your head, neck, and shoulders off the ball. Inhale and reach both arms out shoulder-height in front of your body. Hold this position and exhale, drawing the abs in even more. Inhale and return your arms to your head without moving the upper body. Exhale and lower your head, neck, and shoulders.

Modification: Do the move without the arm extension.

Tracey's Tips

• Do not lower your head as you place your arms back on your head; keep the abs engaged so they're holding you up in the curl before you lower your head.
• Go slowly and hold each part of the move; this intensifies the work in the abs.

3. Down Stretch

Inspiration: Wearing a tight T-shirt

Muscles targeted: Abs, lats, and quads

Reps: 10

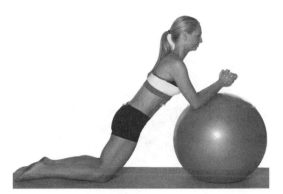 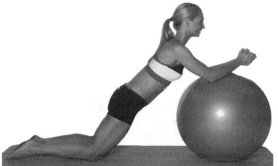

A. Kneel on the floor, resting your forearms on the ball with your shoulders directly over your elbows. Your body should be on a slight incline with your hips pressed forward. (Imagine a diagonal line from the crown of your head to your knees.)

B. Exhale and roll the ball out a few inches so you are balancing on your elbows while keeping your spine in a neutral position. Inhale and return the ball back to the starting position.

Tracey's Tips

• Keep the weight out of your upper body, including the neck and shoulders, by drawing your shoulder blades down the back.
• Pull in your abs the entire time without arching your back.

MOTIVATION FROM TEAM MALLETT

To keep me on track and as a gentle reminder to work out, I kept my favorite pair of pre-pregnancy pants hanging over the chair at the end of my bed.
—*Sally Teiniker, 32, Auckland, New Zealand*

4. Ball Switch

Inspiration: Muffin-top fat burn!

Muscles targeted: Abs and inner thighs

Reps: 10–15

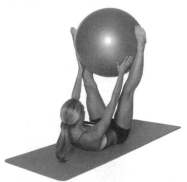

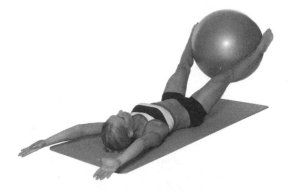

A. Lie on your back with your head, neck, and shoulders off the floor and holding the ball in front of your body. Extend your legs to 90 degrees with your feet in line with your hips.

B. Exhale and place the ball between your legs. Inhale and lower your head, neck, and shoulders with your arms overhead. Keep the ball between your bent legs and lower to 45 degrees (or as far as you can while still maintaining good form).

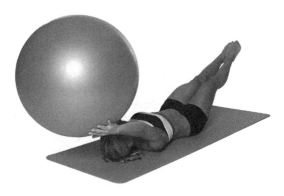

C. Exhale and return your arms and legs up as you lift your head, neck, and shoulders off the floor to grab the ball. Inhale and extend your arms and legs as you lower your head, this time holding the ball over your head.

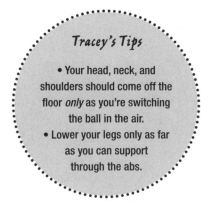

Tracey's Tips

• Your head, neck, and shoulders should come off the floor *only* as you're switching the ball in the air.
• Lower your legs only as far as you can support through the abs.

5. Classic Double Leg Stretch

Inspiration: School reunion!

Muscles targeted: Abs

Reps: 10–12

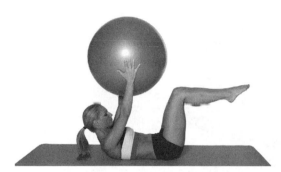

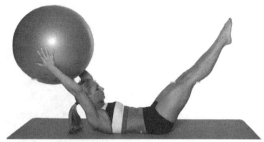

A. Lie on your back with your legs bent at 90 degrees, your shins parallel to the floor, your knees over your hips, and your head, neck, and shoulders off the floor. Focus your eyes toward your belly (keep your chin off your chest) and hold the ball at shoulder height.

B. Inhale and reach your arms overhead until the ball is level with your ears and straighten your legs diagonally. Make sure your abs are drawn in and lower your legs only as far as you can while maintaining good form (a neutral spine). Exhale and bend your arms and knees back to the starting position.

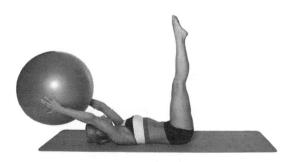

Modification: Keep your head, neck, and shoulders on the floor and your legs straight up toward the ceiling.

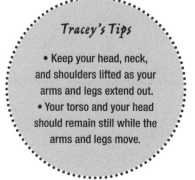

Tracey's Tips

• Keep your head, neck, and shoulders lifted as your arms and legs extend out.
• Your torso and your head should remain still while the arms and legs move.

6. Double Leg Side Lifts

Inspiration: Stand taller with more confidence!

Muscles targeted: Obliques

Reps: 10 each side

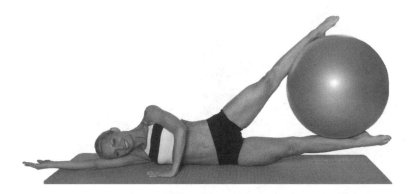

A. Lie on your left side with your legs straight, holding the ball between your ankles, with your hips stacked on top of each other. Your legs should be slightly in front of your torso to reduce strain on the lower back. Your left arm is straight, palm up, with your ear resting on your bicep and your right arm resting on the floor in front of your sternum for support.

B. Inhale to prepare, and exhale as you lift both legs off the floor, drawing the bottom rib closer to the hip bone without shifting your hips back. Inhale and lower your legs.

Tracey's Tip

Watch that your back does not arch. If you feel pain in your back, move your legs further forward.

7. Side Stretch with Ball

Inspiration: Flexible spine.

Purpose: To stretch the obliques and lower back

Reps: Twenty seconds each stretch, twice on each side

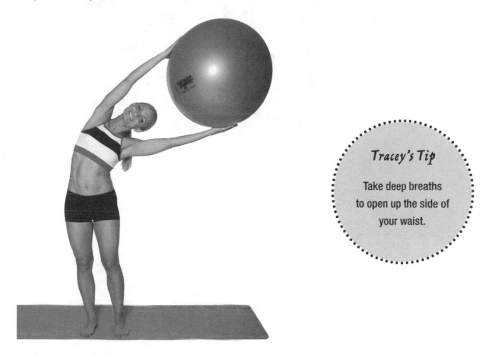

Tracey's Tip

Take deep breaths
to open up the side of
your waist.

A. Stand with legs hip-width apart and hands overhead holding the ball. Make sure your shoulders are pulling away from your ears.

B. Inhale and reach your hands up and over to the right side, keeping your weight equally distributed in both feet and your torso facing forward. Keep your head in line with your spine and looking forward.

Success Story

•••

Sally Teiniker, 32, mother of three, Auckland, New Zealand

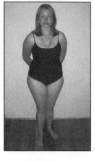
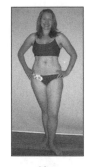
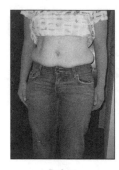
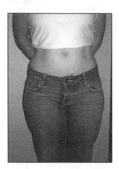

| Before | After | Before | After |

Lost

13 pounds

6 percent body fat

Two dress sizes

4 inches off her waist

3 inches off her hips

1 inch off her thighs

8 inches total

Gained

The figure she had before she became a mom. *I was thrilled to be back into my pre-pregnancy wardrobe at only four months post-partum. With my previous two pregnancies, it took me at least a year and much more effort. I got similar results in this program in just six weeks! This success has made me a happier, more energetic, and confident person.*

• • • • •

Sally Teiniker, a manager for a non-profit organization, kept fit during her third pregnancy. But like any new mom, she still had some weight to lose once her baby was born and wondered if she'd ever see her flat abs again. "I hated carrying around the extra pounds because how I look really affects how I feel about myself," says this 32-year-old from Auckland, New Zealand. Sally needed a healthy way to slim down because she was nursing and didn't want to compromise her milk supply or baby's nutrition. "I also wanted an exercise program that I could do at home and one that I'd actually enjoy," she says. The answer was *Sexy in 6*. "I found it appealing because Tracey has kids, family, and work commitments like I do, and I thought, 'If she can do it, so can I,'" she says.

At first, it was hard for this busy mother of three to put herself first—something that was foreign to her. "But it soon became a habit and was actually a part of the day that I looked forward to," she says. Another change was realizing that breaking a sweat in small increments *can* reap results. "I used to be an all-or-nothing type of person when it came to exercise—if it wasn't at least an hour session in the gym or a 10K run, it didn't seem worth it. Tracey taught me that grabbing whatever time you have, when you have it, could make all the difference. I'm amazed at the results I've gotten in just eighteen minutes a day!"

Sally also had to change her eating habits. As a self-proclaimed carb-based snacker, she learned to incorporate protein at every meal and snack, which kept her feeling fuller. She also reduced her huge portion sizes and cooked healthier dishes. "I love the fact that I can still eat real food and don't have to rely on artificial sweeteners or processed foods to lose weight," she says. "And unlike other diets, I don't have to cook a special meal for me and a separate one for my family." The combination of healthy eating and exercise gave Sally a body she'd never achieved on diets in the past. Being organized was also critical. "When I packed the kids' school lunches in the morning, I prepared my own snacks. Then when I got hungry, I had something healthy and wasn't tempted to reach for the cookies."

SALLY'S STICK-WITH-IT TIP

Put yourself at the top of your to-do list. It's really easy to put the rest of your family first, but the benefits of making yourself a priority for the few weeks it takes to complete the program are just amazing. After that, it becomes a habit you'll be hooked on. Having some dedicated "me" time—even if it's twelve minutes a day—also makes me a better parent to my kids because I feel like I'm doing something for myself.

Even during a difficult week when she had a stomach illness, was up all night with the baby, found out her oldest daughter's camp was cancelled, and realized her TV was broken, Sally stuck with Tracey's program. "In the past, I would have given up at that point and pigged out on chocolate (or worse). But the results I had achieved kept me on track," she says. Plus, the abs she hadn't seen in eons emerged, looking better than ever. "Tracey taught me consistency and that made the biggest difference in my abs. The program didn't ask me to commit hours at a time to my stomach; I only had to do a little bit every day and I got results. It actually felt easy," says Sally. "My favorite exercise was the Side Plank Twist; it was the one that I could easily measure my improvement by. In the beginning I couldn't do it all. But by the end I could do it without any modifications. I have so much more energy to play with the kids and get out of bed in the morning (even if I've been up with the baby all night). I'm a fitter and much happier me."

TRACEY'S TAKE

I first chatted with Sally when she contacted me through my Web site. She was pregnant and had difficulty finding a good comprehensive pregnancy workout. She wanted to stay in the best shape possible while pregnant and have the stamina to keep up with her two other children. I recommended my *3 in 1 Pregnancy System* DVD, which she followed for most of the nine months. Post-partum, doing the *Sexy in 6* program was a natural progression for her. Sally's attitude has always been upbeat and positive, which I truly believe contributes to results. If you think yourself slimmer, you will be slimmer. This is exactly what Sally did, despite a busy family life, a new baby, a job, and a husband. Just look at those abs. That's a sexy stomach for any woman to have, but she got these just five months after having a baby! Wow!

CHAPTER 7

QUICK MIND-BODY BLAST

UNLESS YOU'VE BEEN LIVING UNDER A ROCK, YOU'VE AT least heard of Pilates and yoga. They're popular with professional athletes and dancers, and go in and out of vogue with celebrities, but both disciplines are much more than trends. They have been around for ages. Yoga started about two thousand years ago with an Indian sage named Patanjali. Pilates was the brainchild of Joseph Pilates, a legendary physical trainer, back in the 1920s. Both bring an amazing sense of awareness to your body, teach you how to breathe, sculpt your muscles, and boost your flexibility.

Equally important is the fact that they help you relax and reduce stress. As a busy, working mom in a crazy world, I can vouch for the fact that Pilates and yoga are surefire routes to a calmer you. A new report from Harvard Medical School says that exercises that cause a relaxation response, such as yoga, can help reduce the cumulative negative effects of stress in your body. A relaxation response means that your heartbeat and respiration slow down, your body uses less oxygen and produces less carbon dioxide, and your blood pressure stabilizes.

Yoga and Pilates also improve your posture and strengthen your core (your abdominals and lower back muscles). Yoga may even be the answer to your aching back. Research from the Group Health Cooperative's Center for Health Studies in Seattle had one group of participants with lower back pain take seventy-five-minute yoga classes and practice at home. A second group did seventy-five-minute sessions of aerobic, strengthening, and stretching exercises, and a third group read a self-help book on back pain. In three months, the yogis were better able to do daily activities involving their backs than the other two groups. After six-and-a-

MOTIVATION FROM TEAM MALLETT

The mind-body connection of this program never ceases to amaze me. The measuring tape doesn't show any results yet, neither does the scale; but I feel thinner and that makes me feel more confident. I catch myself stealing glimpses in the mirror and smiling. And I never used to smile while looking in the mirror. I can only imagine how much better I will feel as each week passes.
—Tanya Torforson, 28, Bruderheim, Canada

half months, they had better back-related function and less pain. Plus, fewer people in the yoga group needed to pop pain relievers.

Both Pilates and yoga bring to life parts of the body you never knew existed. My first yoga class was ten years ago. I had just moved to the United States and settled in Los Angeles (where knowing the lotus pose is practically a requirement for residency and yoga mats are accessories). I'd always thought yoga was for lightweights—sort of like the lazy man's exercise. Boy, was I wrong! The moves may look easy, but try holding them for endless periods of time.

The first time I twisted my body into pretzel-poses and downward dogging, I couldn't believe how much strength was required. My legs shook and I thought they'd give out on me any second. I know this may sound like a cliché, but I felt a sense of calmness and control over my body. I felt empowered. I know, you're wondering if you should cue the new age music or "I am woman," but I'm serious.

Today, I do yoga once a week. My favorite type is Hatha yoga, which is often interpreted as the "union" of mind and body. It's a series of physical postures designed to open the many channels of the body—especially the main channel, the spine—so that energy can flow freely and reduce stress. In a world that runs 24/7, where even toddlers multitask, yoga is a fabulous escape.

Then there's Pilates, defined as a series of controlled movements that help to gently condition your body and mind. As a professional dancer for years, Pilates was how I kept my body in top form. Pilates focuses on your core with the goal of creating a strong center and a body that not only moves better but lives better. All exercises require mental concentration along with coordinated breathing. What I love about Pilates is the series of precise movements that focus on symmetry of the body and do not require a lot of repetitions.

> Physical fitness is the first requisite of happiness. Our interpretation of physical fitness is the attainment and maintenance of a uniformly developed body with a sound mind fully capable of naturally, easily, and satisfactorily performing our many and varied daily tasks with spontaneous zest and pleasure.
> —Joseph Pilates

Like yoga, Pilates can be performed almost anywhere—all you need is a mat. You use your own body weight for resistance and there's no bouncing, jarring, or stress on your body, so there's little risk of injury. I love to incorporate moves from both disciplines in the workout routines I create for my clients, my DVDs, and now for you in the Quick Mind-

Body Blast exercises that follow. These moves will energize you as well as soothe and mellow your mind while toning your body. So the next time you're stressed or need a pick-me-up, bypass the potato chips and dip into these Pilates and Yoga inspired moves.

QUICK MIND-BODY BLAST A

ABOUT THE WORKOUT

What It Is: Energizing the body requires the involvement of *all* your muscles. This segment has power moves to tone and build strength in the lower body and core.

How to Do It: Move from one pose to the next in the order given. Start with the right leg, do all the moves in a given Blast, and then repeat on the left.

It Will Take You: Six minutes each segment

You Need: A mat

Contrology [Pilates] is complete coordination of body, mind, and spirit. Through Contrology [Pilates] you first purposefully acquire complete control of your own body, and then through proper repetition of its exercises you gradually and progressively acquire that natural rhythm and coordination associated with all your subconscious activities.

—Joseph Pilates

1. Crescent Lunge

Inspiration: Strong sculpted thighs!

Muscles targeted: Quads, glutes, hamstrings, abs

Hold: Thirty seconds

A. Place your left leg forward about four feet. Bend your left knee into a lunge (thigh parallel to the floor). Extend your back leg straight with knee facing the floor and the toes curled under, balancing on the ball of your foot. Draw your shoulder blades down, away from the ears, and extend your arms overhead, keeping your biceps in line with your ears.

Caution: If you have knee problems, limit how far you bend the front leg.

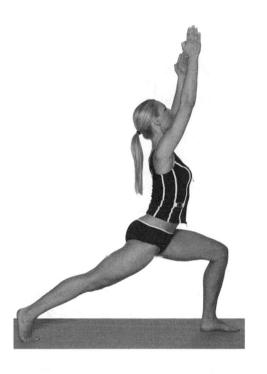

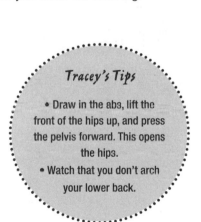

Tracey's Tips

• Draw in the abs, lift the front of the hips up, and press the pelvis forward. This opens the hips.

• Watch that you don't arch your lower back.

2. Warrior Two

Inspiration: Flexible hips and strong legs!

Muscles targeted: Quads, glutes, hamstrings, lats, and abs

Hold: Thirty seconds

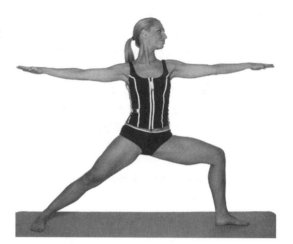

A. From the Crescent Lunge, roll the left hip around to face the left side. Turn the back foot out, keeping it on the floor with the toes pointing forward. (The front heel and instep of the back foot should be in straight line.)

B. Bring your shoulder blades down the back, which activates the lats, and extend your arms straight out to the side at shoulder height.

Caution: Only lunge as far as it feels comfortable and keep the knee *over* the toes.

3. Triangle Pose

Inspiration: Long flexible hamstrings!

Muscles targeted: Quads, glutes, hamstrings, and abs

Hold: Thirty seconds

A. From Warrior Two, reach your left hand toward the front of your left foot and straighten your left leg.

B. Twist your upper body toward the sky, using your abs to rotate your torso further.

C. Extend your right hand up to the sky, with your palms facing away from the body. Focus your eyes on the top hand.

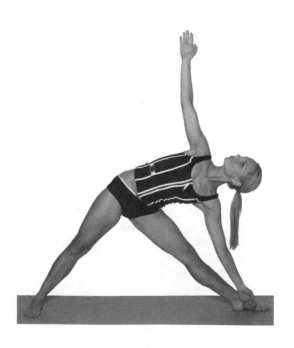

Modification: If your hamstrings aren't super flexible, just hold your shin above the ankle or use a yoga block.

4. Dog Splits

Inspiration: Long scissor-like legs!

Muscles targeted: Hamstrings, quads, and glutes

Hold: Thirty seconds

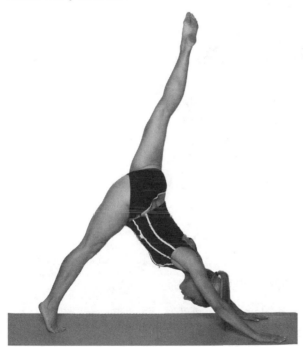

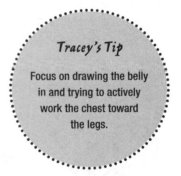

Tracey's Tip

Focus on drawing the belly in and trying to actively work the chest toward the legs.

A. From the Triangle Pose, turn your torso to face forward in a lunge position with your right leg and place your hands on either side of the right foot.

B. Swing your left leg behind your body, extending the spine upward into a downward dog. Rise up onto the ball of the right supporting leg and open the pelvis toward the right side.

5. Plank Position

Inspiration: Strong chiseled core!

Muscles targeted: Chest, shoulders, arms, and abs

Hold: Thirty seconds

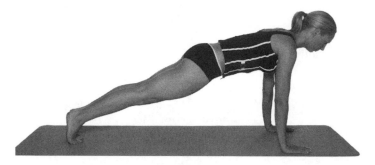

A. Place hands shoulder-width apart with the shoulders directly over the wrists. Extend your legs in a push-up position with toes curled under, resting on the balls of your feet. Imagine pushing away from the floor and activating the lats so there's no sinking in between the shoulder blades. Keep the abs engaged.

6. Standing Head-to-Knee

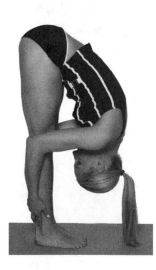

Inspiration: To move with ease!

Muscles targeted: Hamstrings and upper and lower back

Hold: Fifteen seconds

A. Walk the hands toward the feet and gently hold onto the calves, drawing the head toward the knees. Use your upper body strength to pull your body further toward your legs.

Modification: Bend your knees until you find a comfortable position.

7. Standing Spine Extension

Inspiration: Correct posture!

Muscles targeted: Upper spine and hamstrings

Hold: Fifteen seconds

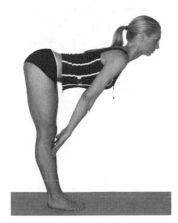

A. Hold onto your shins as you reach your collarbone up toward the ceiling. Roll your shoulder blades down and back toward your hips. Press the weight of your body into the heels of your feet and draw your abs toward your spine.

Modification: Hold onto your knees.

8. Roll-Up

Inspiration: Stress release. Sounds good!

Muscles targeted: Upper and lower spine

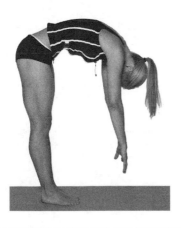

A. Slightly bend your knees and slowly roll up vertebra by vertebra. Contract your abs throughout. End by uncurling your head. Imagine you're breathing space between each vertebra and keep your glutes relaxed.

QUICK MIND-BODY BLAST B

ABOUT THE WORKOUT

What It Is: A short Pilates workout consisting of deep toning exercises. I can't guarantee you'll grow any taller, but it will give the illusion of more height due to better posture and a stronger core.

How to Do It: Perform each exercise once before going on to the next exercise.

It Will Take You: 6 minutes

You Need: A mat

MOTIVATION FROM TEAM MALLETT

I always feel amazing after working out—
especially if I've had a very stressful day at work.
As a result, I feel more positive about everything.
—Laurie Jardin, 43, Ontario, Canada

1.Knee Twists

Inspiration: Teeny, tiny hourglass waist!

Muscles targeted: Obliques

Reps: 20

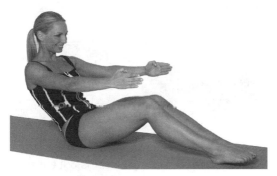 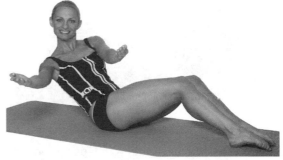

A. Sit tall with your legs bent in front of your body, your inner thighs together, and your hands reaching out in front of you at shoulder height. Roll down your spine until it is in a C shape; engage the abs, and draw your shoulder blades down away from your ears.

B. Inhale as you move your knees to your left side and your arms to your right (eyes should focus on hands). Exhale as you contract the obliques, moving your arms and knees back to the starting position. Repeat, bringing your knees to your right side and arms to your left.

Modification: Just twist the upper body, keeping the lower body still.

Tracey's Tip

Maintain a deep C-curve by drawing in the abdominals, rounding the lower back in a pelvic curl.

2. Chest Lift with Arm Reach in Butterfly Position

Inspiration: Strong pelvic floor!

Muscles targeted: Abs

Reps: 10, working up to 15

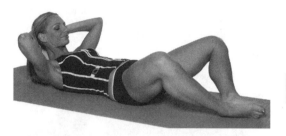 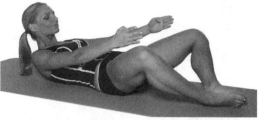

A. Lie on your back with your legs turned out at the hips and the soles of your feet together. (That's the butterfly part.) Place your hands behind your head. Exhale as you draw in your abs and lift your head, neck, and shoulders off the floor, keeping your hips still.

B. Inhale as you reach your arms out toward your feet. Exhale as you draw in your abs (imagine you're scooping out your tummy). Inhale as your upper body stays lifted, bringing your hands back to your head and lowering your head, neck, and shoulders to the floor. Relax the legs so that you do not engage the hip flexors.

Tracey's Tips

• Keep the spine in a neutral position as you lift your upper body.
• If you have tight hamstrings, place two pillows under each knee for gentle support.

3. Single Leg Stretch into Criss-Cross

Inspiration: Unbelievable flat, sculpted midsection. Trust me, this exercise is one of the best for seeing results fast!

Muscles targeted: Abdominals

Reps: 10 single leg stretch and 10 criss-cross

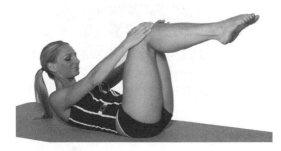

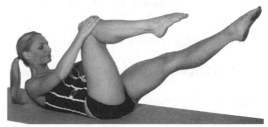

A. Lie on your back with knees bent in line with your hips, knees at a 90-degree angle, and shins parallel to the ceiling. Lift your head, neck, and shoulders off the floor. Rest your hands on your left knee.

B. Exhale, extend your left leg straight, and imagine that you're resisting the right knee, keeping your shin parallel to the floor. Alternate extending legs and switching hands. Continue to exhale as your knee draws toward your chest.

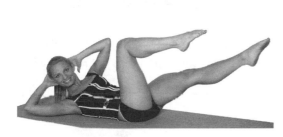

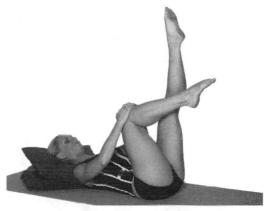

C. Bend your elbows, place your hands behind your head, and rotate your torso toward the opposite hip without moving your pelvis. Aim your shoulder, not your elbow, to the knee. (This helps you achieve true rotation. Just moving your arms is not rotating the body.)

Tracey's Tips

• As you perform the Single Leg Stretch and the knee draws toward the chest, imagine you're resisting the knee with your hands. This creates more resistance for your abs.

• Point your toes and reach out through the big toes. This will add length to the legs and activate all the leg muscles, making the exercise more challenging!

Modification: Place a couple of pillows under your head to elevate your head, neck, and shoulders. This makes sure that all the work is in your abs, not in your neck and shoulders.

Also, as an option you can place your head down on the mat.

4. Double Leg Stretch

Inspiration: Complete core control!

Muscles targeted: Abdominals

Reps: 10

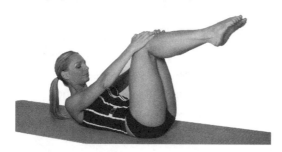

A. Lie on your back with your head, neck, and shoulders off the floor, your hips at a 90-degree angle, and shins parallel to the ceiling. Place your hands on your knees.

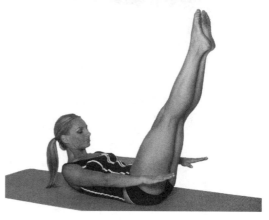

B. Inhale and extend your legs diagonally into the air and reach your hands out toward your feet in line with your hips.

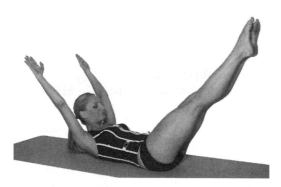

C. Exhale, reach your arms overhead, circle them around, and return them to the sides of your body. Pause and inhale; then exhale and bend your knees back to the starting position.

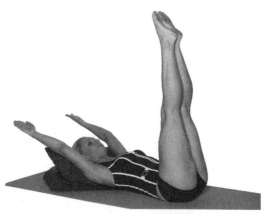

Modification: Add pillows to support the upper body off the floor and extend your legs straight up to the ceiling. Also, as an option you can keep your head on the mat without pillows.

5. Flutter Kicks with Heel Beats

Inspiration: Toned, cellulite-free hamstrings and buns of steel!

Muscles targeted: Glutes, hamstrings, lats, and lower back

Reps: 40

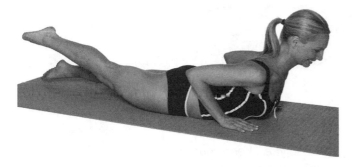

A. Lie on your stomach with your elbows bent and your hands by the sides of your rib cage. Extend your spine, pulling your shoulders down toward your hips.

B. Lift alternate legs off the floor as if you're doing a flutter kick.

Tracey's Tips

• Lift from the hips, so the movement is coming from your butt.
• Your legs should be straight, reaching out through the toes.
• Draw your shoulder blades down toward the hips, activating the lats.

MOTIVATION FROM TEAM MALLETT

*I love your program.
Even during busy times I can easily fit in
six minutes of exercise and I feel less stress after!
—Nancy Compana, 38, Pasadena, California*

6. Pilates Side Leg Series

Inspiration: Pure toned buttocks! Think Jessica Biel.

Muscles targeted: Glutes

Reps: 10 to the side and 10 forward on each leg

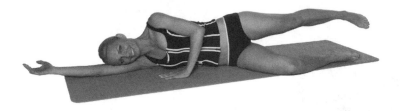

A. Lie on your right side with your ear resting on the bottom outstretched arm. Bend your right leg to 45 degrees. Keep your left leg straight and internally rotate it so that the toe is pointing down to the floor. Lift your left leg up and down 12 inches, keeping your hips stacked and your pelvis completely still.

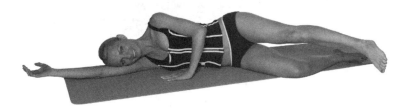

B. Inhale and move your leg forward on a diagonal (be careful not to shift the pelvis), and then return your leg back to the starting position.

Tracey's Tip

Try and relax the entire working leg, forcing the glutes to do all the work without bigger muscles, such as the quads, taking over.

QUICK MIND-BODY BLAST C

ABOUT THE WORKOUT

What It Is: A blend of dynamic and static moves that work the entire body.

How to Do It: Perform each exercise once before going on to the next exercise.

It Will Take You: 6 minutes

You Need: A mat

WHO KNEW?

Wearing high heels tilts your pelvis forward. This shortens your hip flexors and causes your back to arch. Over time, this weakens the lower ab muscles and leaves your lower back feeling tight. The moral: Wear your Jimmy Choo shoes just once or twice a week!

MOTIVATION FROM TEAM MALLETT

After two weeks, my body feels tighter!
Being fit truly is a natural antidepressant!
—Emily Cole, 28, Euless, Texas

1. Side Plank Leg Lift

Inspiration: The ultimate bikini butt! (I do this exercise religiously before going on vacation.)

Muscles targeted: Obliques, abs, glutes, and lats

Reps: 10 each side

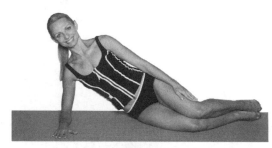 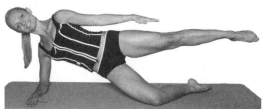

A. Lie on your right side with your knees slightly bent and stacked on top of each other. Rest your right elbow and forearm on the floor, with your shoulder directly in line with your elbow, and place your left arm on your left hip.

B. Exhale and lift your hips off the floor, extending the top leg to hip height. (Keep your shoulder over your elbow at all times.) Lower your hips to the floor gently, without placing too much weight on the hip, and then lift again.

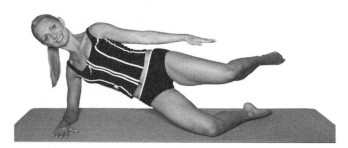

Modification: Keep the top leg bent.

Tracey's Tips

• Draw your shoulder blades down your back, activating the lats and contracting the obliques.
• Keep your hips stacked and facing forward at all times.

2. Dolphin Kick Backs

Inspiration: Sleek and lean thighs!

Muscles targeted: Glutes, hamstrings, obliques, lats, and abs

Reps: 10 each leg

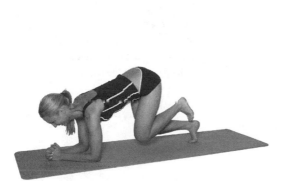

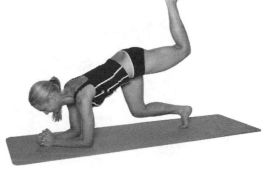

A. Interlace your fingers and rest your forearms on the floor with your knees bent about 10 inches off the floor, so that your shins are parallel to the floor with toes curled under.

B. Keeping your right knee slightly bent, extend your left leg above hip height, leading with the heel toward the ceiling.

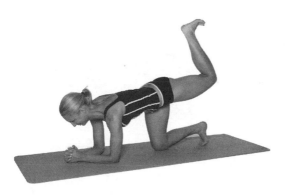

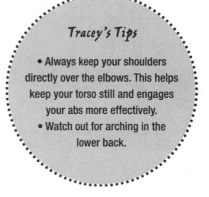

Tracey's Tips

• Always keep your shoulders directly over the elbows. This helps keep your torso still and engages your abs more effectively.

• Watch out for arching in the lower back.

Modification: Keep the supporting knee on the floor.

3. Leg Pull Front

Inspiration: Strong, sexy core and upper body!

Muscles targeted: Abs, upper body, and glutes

Reps: 10 each leg

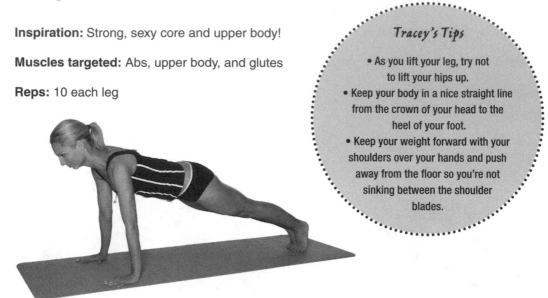

Tracey's Tips

- As you lift your leg, try not to lift your hips up.
- Keep your body in a nice straight line from the crown of your head to the heel of your foot.
- Keep your weight forward with your shoulders over your hands and push away from the floor so you're not sinking between the shoulder blades.

A. Get into a plank position with your hands shoulder-width apart, legs extended, and toes curled under.

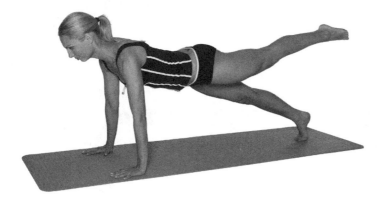

B. Exhale and lift your left leg up without moving the rest of your body. Inhale and lower your leg to the floor.

Modification: Place the opposite knee on the floor for more support.

4. Cat Cow with Leg Extension

Inspiration: Toned physique and a stretched out lower back. Mmmmm heaven!

Muscles targeted: Abs, lats, and glutes

Reps: 5 each side

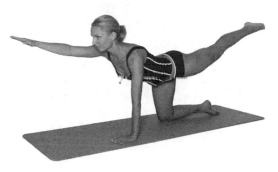
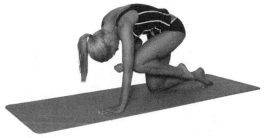

A. Hands shoulder-width apart and knees directly under your hips. Inhale and draw your shoulder blades down the back as you reach your right arm forward at shoulder height and your left leg behind you to hip height, toe and knee pointing downward.

B. Exhale and bend your right arm and left knee toward your chest as you draw your abs in and arch your spine, like an angry cat. Inhale and extend your arm and leg to hip and shoulder height, and repeat.

Modification: Lift only the leg and arm and hold until you have built enough support to add the cat.

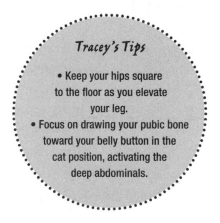

Tracey's Tips

• Keep your hips square to the floor as you elevate your leg.
• Focus on drawing your pubic bone toward your belly button in the cat position, activating the deep abdominals.

5. Chair Position with Heels Elevated

Inspiration: Miniskirt legs. Erin Brockovich, eat your heart out!

Muscles targeted: Quads, hamstrings, calves, and abs

Reps: 10–15

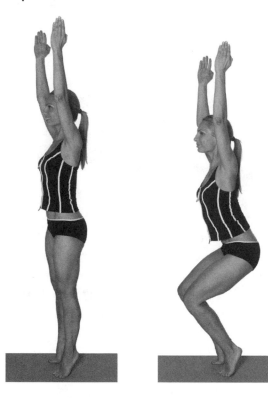

Tracey's Tips

• Extend your spine and heart center to the sky, draw your shoulders away from your ears, and open your chest by aligning your biceps by your ears.
• Pull in your abs to counteract any arching in the lower back.

A. Stand with your feet hip-width apart, balancing on the balls of the feet. Extend your arms over your head so they're in line with your ears.

B. Inhale as you bend your knees and slightly pitch your body forward, drawing your abs in and curling your pelvis under. Exhale and extend your legs, focusing on keeping your heels still. Repeat for a total of 10–15 reps before lowering your heels and standing tall.

Modification: Keep the entire foot planted on the ground.

6. Roll Down

Inspiration: Relaxation (a rare thing but not impossible)

Muscles targeted: Abdominals and hamstrings

Reps: 2

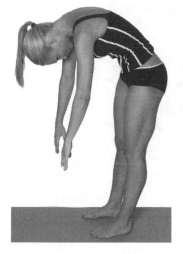

A. Stand with your feet hip-width apart and your hands by the sides of your body. Exhale as you contract your abs and draw your chin toward your chest. Roll down toward the floor through the spine and pause slightly, feeling the stretch in your hamstrings and lower back.

B. Inhale. Then exhale, unrolling the spine, stacking each vertebra, with the head being the last to uncurl.

QUESTION FROM TEAM MALLETT

I've heard that Pilates and yoga may help with lower back pain. If so, how?

Pilates is great for alleviating lower back pain because the exercises are centered on conditioning the core. The deepest of these muscles is the transverse abdominal, which is like a corset around the waist; it stabilizes and protects the spine. The only true way to activate these muscles is through forcefully exhaling and drawing in the abdominal wall at the same time. Pilates teaches us how to activate this muscle and continuously use it to stabilize the spine throughout all exercises. Yoga stretches out tight muscles such as the hamstrings, which attach to the pelvis. This helps the spine move more freely in its natural state, alleviating pressure in the lower back.

Success Story

···

Alison Fukomoto, 29, Santa Monica, California

Lost

13 pounds

4 percent body fat

1 dress size

2 inches off her arms

2½ inches off her waist

1 inch off her hips

2 inches off her thighs

7½ total inches lost

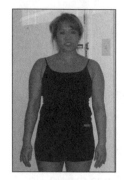

Before

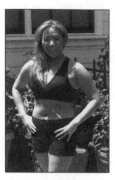

After

Gained

A healthy lifestyle that she can stick with forever. *All around, this program has been a good change for me. I've learned to eat better and fit workouts and a healthy diet into my crazy, professional life. I feel so much better about myself.*

Alison Fukomoto, 29, knew her life as a busy, single professional woman was taking a toll on her body. As a child and teenager, Alison stayed slim by being active and playing sports. But thanks to ten- to twelve-hour workdays as a project manager for an IT company and a daily three-hour commute, her activity level decreased and the pounds crept onto her 5-foot 1-inch frame. Although she'd tried some trendy diets over the last three years, she'd lost and regained 10 to 15 pounds several times. "I was sluggish and always tired. I didn't like how I looked and I didn't feel good about myself," she says. "I wanted to get exercise into my lifestyle, along with better eating habits, but wasn't sure how to do it without feeling deprived."

Before the program, Alison didn't eat breakfast—unless you count gulping down a double espresso from Starbucks. Lunch and dinner were often high-fat, high-calorie fast-food meals such as pizza, pasta, and sandwiches. Another big problem were the fattening, unhealthy snacks that were all too plentiful at her office. "Comfort foods were available for those of us who were working long hours," says Alison, who was "hooked" on Cheetos and cookies. She rarely exercised—despite the fact that she's a certified Pilates instructor.

All that changed when she joined Team Mallett. "Any other exercise programs and diets I'd tried made me feel like I was giving things up. This program was flexible and had the perfect amount of push for motivation and ease," she says. The biggest difference this time? "Tracey's program is a new food *lifestyle*—not a short-term diet—and it's something I actually enjoy," she says. "I *love* food and I'm completely content with what I'm eating on this plan—unlike diets I've been on—so I know this won't change. I've found healthy, convenient ways to have really good meals and snacks."

Now, instead of going out to eat, Alison eats multigrain cereal with flaxseed and berries and non-fat milk for breakfast and cooks a lot more. When she does go to a restaurant, she has learned to make better choices. She has also discovered food substitutes that don't make her feel like she's sacrificing anything. "I found a great garlic mustard to replace mayonnaise on my sandwiches and I cook with ground turkey instead of ground pork. I also eat low-fat and non-fat dairy—such as sour cream and milk—and fruit for snacks." Planning ahead means she's no longer a regular in her office's snack room. "I can't eat junk food anymore. It actually makes me sick," says Alison. Her new food plan has become such a natural part of her life that even during weeks where twelve- to fourteen-hour workdays were the norm, Alison kept the pounds at bay. "Usually, that's when my eating goes downhill, but I maintained my healthy habits and I'm so proud of that," she says.

As for exercise, Alison is back on track. "Tracey's workout program fits into my life," she says. "I have extra energy when I work out in the morning and sleep better when I do it at night," says Alison, who was so

ALISON'S STICK-WITH-IT TIP

Be consistent. If you just do that little bit once a day or once every two days, you will lose weight.

energized by her workouts that cutting caffeine out of her diet was a cinch. "Doing the exercises also helped me de-stress, and I discovered the connection between my mind and body. Knowing that you can work parts of your body more by concentrating gave me something to focus on (instead of letting my mind wander) and I actually finished my workouts feeling more relaxed as a result." In addition to doing Tracey's program, Alison dusted off her Pilates certification and now teaches once a week. "The best compliment I got was that I was shrinking," she says. "My clothes fit better and I truly feel healthy."

TRACEY'S TAKE

I've have known Alison for about six years, and I've never seen her look so good. She has a constant smile on her face. Alison is a typical businesswoman expected to put in ten- to twelve-hour days. (I get tired just thinking about her schedule!) She needed a program that was easy and quick to fit that insane life. Seeing results in the first week was the boost she needed to get hooked. I have a tremendous amount of admiration for Alison: She stuck with the plan and finally got the confidence boost to finally teach Pilates after a three-year break. I'm proud of her!

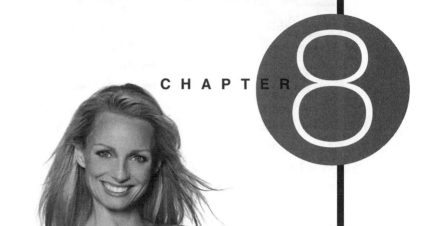

CHAPTER 8

QUICK
CARDIO
BLAST

EXERCISE HAS LOTS OF BENEFITS. SO WHAT'S MY FAVORITE? A round, lifted butt? Flat abs after two pregnancies? The ability to keep up with my energetic toddler? Nope. I *do* love all those things, but reaping those rewards takes time. I like instant gratification, and exercise immediately lifts my spirits. Experts attribute it to endorphins: mood-boosting feel-good chemicals that get released in your brain thanks to exercise.

Not to get too technical, but these endorphins attach themselves to special receptors in the brain and spinal cord to stop pain messages. These are the same receptors that respond to morphine. (Yes, morphine!) The result is a mental lift, not only while you're breaking a sweat, but afterward. See why cardio is my favorite activity? I'm an endorphin junkie. It keeps you sane, reduces stress, and leaves your body feeling refreshed and energized afterwards.

A good cardio session—whether it's running, hiking, or biking—is well-deserved "me time." I can't tell you how many times working out just for a few minutes has saved the day. I can block out kids crying, clients obsessing, and my cell phone ringing. Suddenly my husband's work papers all over the floor aren't so annoying. My head is clear.

And I'm not the only one. Research has shown that exercise may be a great antidepressant. A twelve-week study at UT Southwestern Medical Center found that symptoms of mild to moderate depression decreased by an amazing 50 percent in people who did just thirty minutes of moderately intense aerobic exercise on the treadmill or stationary bike three to five times a week. Researchers say these results are comparable to some studies in which participants used antidepressants or engaged in cognitive therapy. And even those who did low-intensity aerobics reaped results, with symptoms decreasing by about 30 percent. "Exercise may work by changing levels of [brain chemicals], like serotonin, and such changes have been reported to help improve symptoms of depression," explains study author Madhukar Trivedi, M.D., associate professor of psychiatry and head of the depression and anxiety disorders program at UT Southwestern Medical Center. "Numerous effective treatments for depression are available, yet many people don't seek help because of the negative social stigma still associated with the disease. Exercise may offer

WHO KNEW?

Endorphin is Greek for *the morphine within,* the pain-relief chemicals produced naturally in the body during exercise.

a viable alternative." Trivedi's other research has shown that regular workouts may boost the effectiveness of antidepressant medications called selective serotonin reuptake inhibitors (SSRI) such as Prozac, Paxil, Zoloft, Wellbutrin, and Effexor. So give yourself an exercise prescription any time your mood takes a nosedive. Try it, you'll be hooked!

Clients often ask me, "What time of day is best to do cardio?" The short answer? Any time. Most of us live go-go-go crazy lives, so if you have a moment to work out, no matter how small, grab it. Team Mallett member Emily Cole is a single, working mom who often did her workouts at 2 in the morning because that was the only time she had. However, if you're lucky enough to be able to choose when you do cardio, think about how you feel throughout the day and try to schedule it for when you're the most energetic.

That said, I'm convinced that you're more likely to stick with your program if you do it in the morning because you get it over with. Over. Done. Kaput. Cross that baby off your to-do list. If I get in my morning workout, I eat a good breakfast, load up on fruits and veggies, and drink my eight glasses of water. I just start off feeling so good, I want to ride that high all day. But if I skip my early morning exercise, you'll find me walking around feeling sluggish, munching on my kids' leftover pizza crusts and pancakes, and leaving my water bottle behind. Morning workouts set a healthy tone for the rest of your day.

I know it's hard to kick your butt out of your lovely warm bed in the morning, but just think what a buzz you will have *all* day knowing that chore is over. (When I'm all toasty and warm under the covers and thinking of blowing off my workout, I tell myself, "A few more minutes of sleep

Tracey's Tip

I have a little something I tell myself when my motivation lags: "I always finish a workout feeling better than when I started." Okay, it's not up there with the most memorable words in history, but it's simple and true. Try saying that when the last thing you want to do is work out, and I promise it will help.

MOTIVATION FROM TEAM MALLETT

The first time I tried this cardio workout I loved it. It made my treadmill experience the best ever! It went by so quickly and I truly felt like I got a great workout without the typical boredom of a treadmill. I feel great and energized and I want to thank you!
—*Melanie Wyckoff, 33, Vancouver, Washington*

isn't going to do much. But a few minutes of exercise can change my whole day—and my body." It works every time!) Otherwise, by the time evening comes around, so many things can stop you from working out. Excuses abound, and who cares about the treadmill when you're tired, hungry, and stressed? Eventually, when you're glowing, energized, and less stressed, exercise will develop into a healthy addiction—and there's nothing wrong with being addicted to feeling good.

Here's an added push to make like an early bird. Working out in the morning burns slightly more fat. Early in the morning before you eat, your levels of muscle and liver glycogen (stored carbs) are low. Why? Well, say you eat dinner at 6 p.m. and don't eat breakfast until 7 a.m. That's thirteen hours without food. During this overnight fast, your levels of glycogen slowly decline to provide glucose for various bodily functions that go on even while you sleep. As a result, you wake up in the morning with depleted glycogen for energy. This is your body's primary and preferred energy source. But when this is in short supply after that thirteen-hour fast, it forces your body to tap into its secondary or reserve energy: body fat. (However, if this makes you light-headed or nauseous, you may need a very light snack such as a hard-boiled egg, half a protein shake, or a small apple with a teaspoon of peanut butter at least thirty minutes before you work out.)

The big key with cardio is finding something you enjoy doing. Researchers at the University of Michigan found that women who break a sweat just to lose weight or become more toned do almost 40 percent less exercise and walk 2.5 times less than those who work out because it reduces stress, energizes them, increases their well-being, or is an activity they like. Finding something you like to do isn't hard today when there are so many options, such as cardio machines at the gym (treadmill, elliptical, stationary bike), walking, running in the great outdoors, or simply working out to your DVDs at home.

INTERVAL TRAINING

The *Sexy in 6* cardio workouts are designed around interval training, which has been proven to boost calorie burn in shorter amounts of time. For busy women, this is the perfect way to get more bang for your workout buck. Interval training is when you alternate short, fast bursts of intensive exercise with slower, less intense intervals of exercise as opposed to just running, biking, or walking at one steady pace. Athletes and sports teams have been using this training method for decades and the results are more power and speed. But it's also an amazing workout for those of us who aren't looking to win medals but are longing to slim down, tone up, and get in better shape.

Researchers at McMaster University in Hamilton, Ontario, found that study participants who did cycling sprint intervals for just two and a half hours a week reaped the same fitness benefits as cyclists who biked for more than ten hours at a moderate and steady pace. One reason why interval training is so effective is that it works both your aerobic and anaerobic systems. During the short bursts of high-intensity effort, your body uses the energy stored in its muscles (glycogen). During the recovery phase (the lower-intensity segments), your heart and lungs work together to break down the lactic acid your body has built up during high-intensity segments. It's in this phase that the aerobic system is in control, using oxygen to convert stored carbohydrates into energy. In time, your muscles develop a higher tolerance to the build-up of lactate and your heart muscle gets stronger.

On the other hand, if you just do your cardio at one steady pace, eventually your body gets used to the workout, gets more efficient at it, and then burns fewer calories while you do it. Mixing intervals into your workout helps stop this from happening. For example, say you're running at 5 miles per hour (mph) for three minutes and then for thirty seconds you sprint like crazy, maybe somewhere around 7 mph. You've just given your body a little shock and challenged it. Your heart rate soars for that thirty seconds and even for part of the slower-paced interval that fol-

MOTIVATION FROM TEAM MALLETT

Interval training is great. After doing one interval run on the treadmill as she suggested, I really felt a surge of energy, like I'd amped up my metabolism. I also am pleased to see that doing just twelve minutes of the total body circuit and/or abs can make a difference—on days when I can't get out and run or go to the gym, I feel like I have a great option to do something that makes me feel better.

—*Erin Lamb, 37, San Marino, California*

lows. Plus, knowing that you have to go all-out only for a short period of time makes it a lot easier to do it. I mean, we can do *anything* for thirty seconds, right?

I know this is all very science-y and technical, but all you need to know is this: Overall, interval training boosts your performance by enabling your muscles to use oxygen more efficiently. This allows you to work harder and burn more calories and fat.

More results for less time? This busy mom will take it! Just make sure that you introduce high-intensity intervals slowly, even if you're an experienced exerciser. Start with short intervals (such as thirty-second fast-paced intervals with three to four minutes of slow-paced ones), and then progress to shorter steady-state cycles and longer intervals. Every workout is different, so switch it up and, I promise, you'll never get bored.

THE DREADED PLATEAU

The plateau is when you're eating and exercising the same as before, but for some reason the scale won't budge. To say it's annoying is an understatement. This is usually when frustration sets in and, even worse, when some people get so fed up they throw in the towel. Don't! Instead, look at your plateau in a positive way. When you're stuck at a weight after doing so well on the plan, it means your metabolism is doing its job. You're probably rolling your eyes at me again, but it's true. Your metabolism is reflecting your newer, slimmer body, a body that doesn't require as many calories as before.

Eventually, you *will* come to a point where the energy output equals the energy input and the result is the good old plateau. To push yourself off that plateau and keep your weight loss chugging along, we need this equation to be negative. That's okay. It just means that you may have to

MOTIVATION FROM TEAM MALLETT

After just three weeks, I'm up to thirty minutes of intervals on the elliptical, up from a very difficult ten minutes six weeks ago.
—*Rachel Cronnin, 37, Cincinnati, Ohio*

reevaluate your workout program and eating plan. Maybe it's time to add an extra cardio session or cut out those extra treats. I'd rather add more exercise to cause a deficit; this can be as simple as working out at a harder intensity or adding another Quick Total-Body Blast.

Remember to be realistic about your weight. It's easy to get carried away, especially after all the amazing compliments you'll get from friends and family. It may push you to go further than you need to. It's important to know that there's a fine line between looking healthy and looking too thin.

GETTING STARTED

It's important to remember to monitor your exertion in my cardio segments with the RPE chart in chapter 1. Listen to your body and, with practice, you will be able to safely monitor your heart rate and push yourself even harder.

TRACEY'S INTERVAL TRAINING SAFETY TIPS

1. Always make sure your body is warmed up before going into an interval. Try walking or running for at least a few minutes before starting the intervals.
2. Listen to your body and work within your own limits. Even though an interval is high intensity, you should still be able to string words together.
3. Set reasonable goals. For example, if you're new to this form of activity, walk for three minutes and then run for one minute, building up gradually.
4. Slow your pace down considerably in the rest period to give your body time to recover.
5. Train on a flat, even surface and slowly introduce hills on some days to switch your workouts.

QUICK TOTAL-BODY BLAST A

ABOUT THE WORKOUT

What It Is: A total-body cardio interval workout.

How To Do It: Start with a one-minute cardio interval and then do two sets of the first exercise. Next, do another one-minute cardio interval and then do two sets of exercise two. March in place for a few minutes between Blasts until you build up your strength to perform them without a break.

It Will Take You: Six minutes per segment

You Need: 3–5 pound weights are needed. I suggest you start off with 3-pound dumbbells and progress to heavier weights as the exercises get easier. You will be working the upper and lower body simultaneously.

CARDIO MUST DO'S

• Have water and a towel nearby and drink regularly before, during, and after the workout.

• Listen to your body. You should always be able to hold a conversation. If you can't chat, chances are you're working too hard and should slow down your pace.

• If at any time during a workout you start to feel nauseous, lightheaded, or short of breath, take a break. If this continues to happen, *refrain* from exercise and consult your physician a.s.a.p.

QUICK TOTAL-BODY CARDIO BLAST A

Warm-up: Walk in place for a few minutes or walk up and down the stairs to slowly warm up your body and elevate your heart rate. Start the first interval a little slower than the others, making sure you're totally warmed up.

1. One-Minute Interval: Bouncing Ball Shuffle

Inspiration: Getting your heart rate up to burn maximum calories!

Muscles targeted: Glutes, hamstrings, and quads

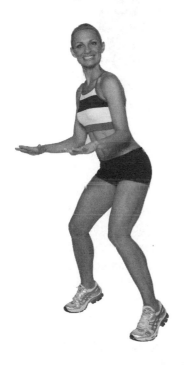

Tracey's Tips

• Keep your body level at all times; imagine you're balancing a plate of fruit on top of your head.
• Focus on pushing off the outside leg with the glute (for example, push off the right leg if traveling left and vice versa).
• Keep both knees bent and try to take wide strides to the side (depending on your workout space).
• Lean with your heel as you move sideways; this ensures that your toes stay pointing forward.

A. Stand with your feet shoulder-width apart, knees slightly bent, and your hands in front of your torso pretending to hold a ball.

B. Shuffle from side to side (four side steps in both direction) for a count of four each way, pretending to bounce a ball.

2. Side Lunge with Row

Inspiration: A sculpted back and sleek thighs.

Muscles targeted: Quads, hamstrings, glutes, shoulders, and mid-upper back

Reps: 10 twice through on each side

Weights: 3- to 5-pound dumbbells

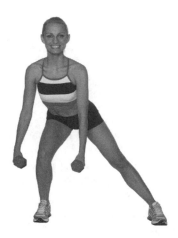 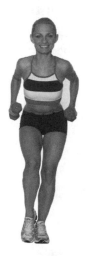

A. Stand tall with legs together and slightly bent. Your arms should be by the sides of your body.

Inhale and step out to the right side with your right foot into a side lunge, the knee and toes facing forward. Twist your upper body and reach your arms toward the bent knee.

B. Exhale and push off your bent right leg, dragging it to meet your left leg. At the same time, bring your shoulder blades together and your elbows behind your body into a row. Your upper body should be pitched forward slightly.

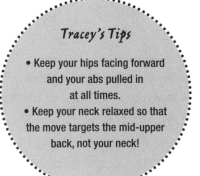

Tracey's Tips

• Keep your hips facing forward and your abs pulled in at all times.
• Keep your neck relaxed so that the move targets the mid-upper back, not your neck!

3. One-Minute Interval: Split Lunge Cross Country

Inspiration: Burn, burn, burn, calories, calories, calories!

Muscles targeted: Quads, hamstrings, glutes, calves, and obliques

Reps: As many as you can do in one minute, keeping good form

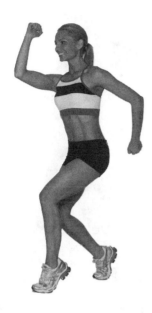

A. Start with your left leg in front with both knees bent and hips facing forward. Bend your right arm in front of your face and bend your left arm behind the body in opposition to the legs (that is, an exaggerated power walk).

B. Jump up into the air, switching legs as you jump so that you land with your left leg in front and your arms in opposition. Repeat, alternating legs, for one minute.

Modification: If you have knee or back problems, do not jump. Switch the legs without leaving the floor.

Tracey's Tips

• Twist the torso toward the front leg as you move your arms to target the waist.
• Big arm movements make you work harder and elevate your heart rate.

4. Chopping Wood

Inspiration: Bye-bye, muffin top! (Keep repeating it like a chant)

Muscles targeted: Shoulders, obliques, glutes, hamstrings, and quads

Reps: 10 twice through on each side

Weights: 3- to 5-pound dumbbell

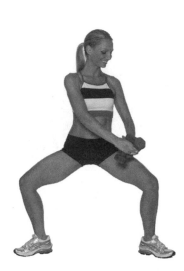 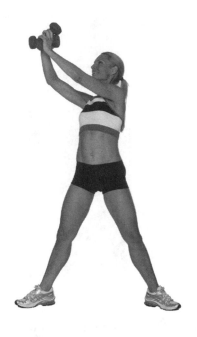

A. Stand with your legs shoulder-width apart, turned out at the hips and knees bent (toes pointing to the corners of the room). Slightly bend your arms, holding both weights together resting on the left hip.

B. Exhale and extend both knees as you rotate your torso toward the right side. At the same time, move your arms diagonally across the body toward the right shoulder. Inhale and bend your knees, returning your arms back to your left hip (the starting position). Focus on your hands at all times.

Modification: If the weight of two dumbbells is too heavy, perform the exercise with just one dumbbell.

Tracey's Tip

Try and keep your hips facing forward and rotate from the waist, which makes the obliques work harder.

QUICK TOTAL-BODY CARDIO BLAST B

Note: If this is your first Blast, you need to warm up gently by either marching in place or walking up and down the stairs until you feel ready to start.

1. One-Minute Interval: Knee Repeater Ab Crunch

Inspiration: Tight, toned abs and a good thigh Blast!

Muscles targeted: Quads, hamstrings, calves, and abs

Reps: As many as you can do on each leg in thirty seconds, keeping good form

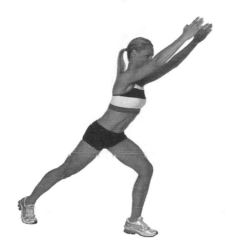
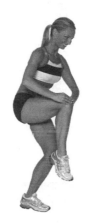

A. Start in a deep lunge with your left leg in front of your right. Your left knee should be over your toes and your right leg should be extended behind your body with your toes curled under, resting on the ball of the foot. Extend both arms forward at shoulder height.

B. Bring your right knee and arms toward your chest as you contract your abs. Keep your left leg bent, forcing the quads to work harder.

Tracey's Tips

• Resist your knee with your arms and focus on contracting the abs as you bring your knee toward your chest.
• Keep at one level and try not to go up and down.

2. Hamstring Curls with Triceps Extensions

Inspiration: Zap the cellulite and tone the arm flab. What could be better than that?

Muscles targeted: Hamstrings, triceps, glutes, and abs

Reps: 10 each leg twice through on each side

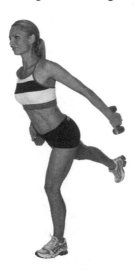
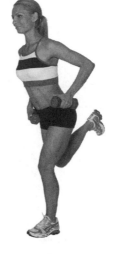

A. Stand on your left leg (slightly bent) with your right leg lifted behind your body about two feet off the floor. Pitch your upper body slightly forward from the hips and rest your right hand on your right hip. The left arm is extended straight behind the body with the palm facing toward the body.

Modification: Hold onto a chair or wall for balance.

B. Inhale and bend your elbow and knee toward your body at the same time. Exhale and extend your arm and leg back to starting position, trying to keep the upper leg and arm still. After finishing reps, switch arms and legs.

Tracey's Tips

• As you move your heel toward the butt, keep the thigh as still as possible and contract the hamstring.
• Contract the abs for support and balance.
• Watch that your lower back does not arch.

3. One-Minute Interval: Jump Rope (or Pretend to Jump Rope)

Inspiration: To be able skip rope without tripping. (I'm still trying.)

Muscles targeted: Quads, hamstrings, calves, and arms

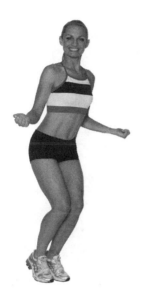

A. Stand with feet shoulder-width apart and arms by your sides holding onto a jump rope (or pretending to).

B. Spring from one foot to the other holding onto the skipping rope or pretending to. Jumping rope is a great calorie burn, not just for the kids!

MOTIVATION FROM TEAM MALLETT

I love the elliptical interval workout. I'm much more motivated having Tracey talk me through the exercise—rather than just jumping on and doing a preset program. It's great to have someone pushing me to the edge of my abilities instead of sitting back and taking it easy. And it's good to have someone to curse at when things get tough!
—Sally Teiniker, 32, Auckland, New Zealand

4. Squat Lift with Lateral Side Lifts

Inspiration: Glute dents (you know, those cute dimples on the side of your derriere). In plain English, a better-looking bottom!

Muscles targeted: Quads, glutes, abs, and shoulders

Reps: 10 twice through each side

Weights: 3- or 5-pound dumbbell

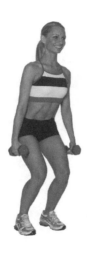 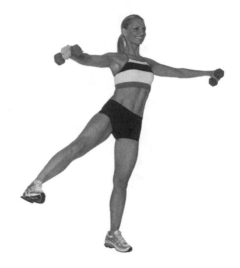

A. Stand with your feet shoulder-width apart and your knees bent in line with your toes in a squat position. Bend your arms slightly by the sides of your body.

B. Extend both knees and contract your abs for balance. Leading with your heel, lift your right leg off the floor to the side of your body without hiking your hips. Your knee and toe should be facing forward. At the same time, open your arms to the sides of your body at shoulder height, leading with your elbows. Keep hips level.

Modifications: Transfer your leg to a toe resting on the floor; don't lift your leg. If you have shoulder problems, do the exercise without weights.

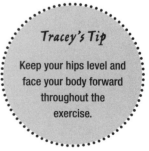

Tracey's Tip

Keep your hips level and face your body forward throughout the exercise.

QUICK TOTAL-BODY CARDIO BLAST C

Note: If this is your first Blast, you need to warm up gently by either marching in place or walking up and down the stairs until you feel ready to start.

1. One-Minute Interval: Double Pulse Squats with Jump

Inspiration: Strong, powerful legs!

Muscles targeted: Quads, hamstrings, glutes, and calves

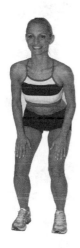

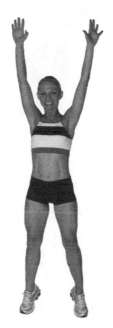

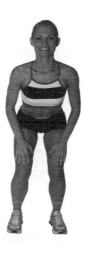

A. Stand with your feet shoulder-width apart, your knees slightly bent, and your arms by the sides of your body. Bend your knees, keeping your weight in your heels. Then pulse up and down two times.

Modification: Keep at least one foot on the ground and step up and over.

B. Lift both legs off the floor and spring up and over, back into a squat position, with both arms reaching overhead. (Imagine you're jumping over a small hedge.)

C. Repeat with another double pulse in the squat position, jumping in the opposite direction. Repeat this for one minute.

Tracey's Tips

• Use the strength in your legs to propel you up in the air.
• Keep the image of a small hedge underneath you. This will inspire you to jump higher.

2. Flamingo with Biceps Lift

Inspiration: To be able to balance on one leg and not fall over!

Muscles targeted: Quads, glutes, hamstrings, biceps, and shoulders

Reps: 10 twice through on each leg

Weights: 3- to 5-pound dumbbell

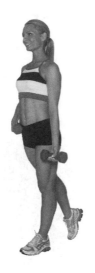 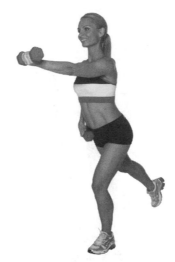 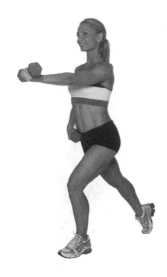

A. Stand on your left leg, with your right leg extended behind you resting on a toe. Rest your right arm on your hip. Place your left arm by the side of your body with your palm facing forward.

B. Inhale, bend your left leg, and extend your right leg off the floor to a comfortable height (your knee should stay in line with the first and second toe). At the same time, lift your left arm to shoulder height. Exhale and return to the starting position.

Modifications: Don't lift the leg behind you; just drag the toe along the floor. Hold onto a chair or a wall for support.

Tracey's Tips

• Stand tall and focus on contracting the core for balance and support.
• Press down into the heel of the foot as your extend your leg. This works your hamstrings and glutes more efficiently.

3. One-Minute Interval: Chuga, Choo, Choo

Inspiration: To be like a kid again and just have fun!

Muscles targeted: Quads, hamstrings, and calves

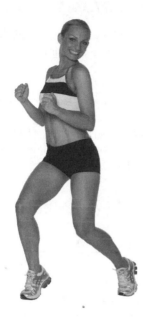

> **Tracey's Tip**
>
> Don't be afraid to really bend the knees and travel forward with big steps to elevate the heart.

A. With your knees bent, step to the right side with your right leg and jump, bringing the left leg to meet the right leg. Repeat with the other leg, alternating sides. Keep your elbows bent and circle your arms down and up with the side steps (like a train). Travel forward and backward.

Modification: Keep one foot on the floor at all times.

MOTIVATION FROM TEAM MALLETT

I was so sore after doing my cardio yesterday!!
But I got out of bed this morning to do the Quick Cardio Blast
and found I had more energy than I thought!
—Alison Fukomoto, 29, Santa Monica, California

4. Plank with Row

Inspiration: Tone the torso, abs, and back all at the same time!

Muscles targeted: Abs, lats, and mid-upper back

Reps: 10 twice through each side

Weights: 3- to 5-pound dumbbell

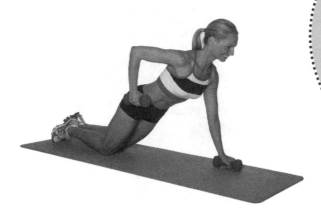

Tracey's Tips

• Keep the whole body still except for the working arm.
• Imagine that the shoulder blades are drawing down the back toward the hips. You will feel the sides of the back (lats) working more efficiently.
• Don't sink in the middle of the shoulder blades. Imagine pushing away from the floor, engaging your upper back muscles.

A. Holding dumbbells shoulder-width apart on the floor, get into a bent-knee push-up position (so you're balancing on the weights and your knees). Move your shoulders directly over your hands and contract your abs. Think of a straight diagonal line from the crown of your head to your knee.

B. Bend your right elbow behind your body and draw your right shoulder blade to the middle of your back. Lower your arm down to the floor, maintaining a still torso by contracting your abs for support.

Modification: Position yourself on all fours with your shoulders directly over your hands and your hips directly over your knees.

COOL DOWN

Finish with a gentle march in place for a few minutes, gradually bringing your heart rate down. Take deep breaths.

BONUS CARDIO WORKOUTS

I know that finding time for cardio is almost impossible and is usually the last thing that most of us want to do. These short workouts are perfect for beginners. Start with the six-minute workouts and then progress to the thirty-minute workouts as you gradually build strength.

Tracey's Tips

• Warm up for five minutes at 0.0 incline and 3.5–5.0 mph. Don't blow off your warm-up. You always need to start your workout at a steady, moderate pace, gradually warming up the body so that oxygen can get to those working muscles.
• Have water and a towel nearby and drink regularly throughout the workout.
• Hold onto the treadmill for support if you are a beginning exerciser or don't have the best balance. Pull in your abs and stand nice and tall. Your hands are there purely for support, so try not to put too much weight into your arms.
• For those who need no support, think of your arms as power levers, rotating your torso as you walk or run. This tiny action works deep into the core—especially the obliques—so you're whittling your middle and doing cardio at the same time.
• Take deep breaths and you will start to feel your heart rate elevating. By the end of the five minutes you should feel comfortable but slightly breathless. Remember that you should be able to hold a conversation throughout this workout.

THE TREADMILL

SIX-MINUTE WORKOUT: TREADMILL

0.00–1.00	WARM-UP WALK AT 3.5 MPH	RPE 4
2.00–3.00	PROGRESS TO A SLOW JOG AT 5.0 MPH	RPE 5
3.00–3.30	INTERVAL JOG AT 6.0 MPH	RPE 6–7
3.30–4.30	JOG AT 5.0 MPH	RPE 5
4.30–5.00	INTERVAL JOG AT 6.5 MPH	RPE 7
5.00–5.30	JOG AT 5.0 MPH	RPE 5
5.30–6.00	COOL DOWN WALK AT 3.5 MPH	RPE 3–4

THIRTY-FIVE-MINUTE WORKOUT: TREADMILL

0.00–1.00	START WALKING AT 3.5 MPH	RPE 4
1.00–5.00	WARM-UP JOG AT 3.5–5.0 MPH	RPE 5
5.00–6.00	INCLINE INTERVAL AT 0.5 INCLINE AND 6.0 MPH	RPE 6–7
6.00–9.00	RECOVERY AT 0.0 INCLINE AND 5.5 MPH	RPE 5–6
9.00–10:00	INCLINE INTERVAL AT 0.5 INCLINE AND 6.0–7.0 MPH	RPE 7
10.00–13.00	RECOVERY AT 0.0 INCLINE AND 5.5 MPH	RPE 5–6
13:00–14.00	INCLINE INTERVAL AT 0.5 INCLINE AND 6.0–7.0 MPH	RPE 7
14:00–17:00	RECOVERY AT 0.0 INCLINE AND 5.0–5.5 MPH	RPE 5–6
17.00–20:00	INCLINE INTERVAL AT 0.5 INCLINE AND 6.5–7.5 MPH	RPE 7–8
20:00–23:00	RECOVERY AT 0.0 INCLINE AND 5.0–5.5 MPH	RPE 5–6
23.00–24:00	INCLINE INTERVAL AT 0.5 INCLINE AND 6.5–7.5 MPH	RPE 7–8
24:00–27:00	RECOVERY AT 0.0 INCLINE AND 5.0–5.5 MPH	RPE 5–6
27.00–28:00	INCLINE INTERVAL AT 0.5 INCLINE AND 6.0–7.0 MPH	RPE 7–8
28:00–31:00	RECOVERY AT 0.0 INCLINE AND 5.0–55 MPH	RPE 5–6
31:00–35:00	COOL DOWN AT 3.5–4.5 MPH	RPE 3–4

Gradually start bringing your heart rate down until you feel your heartbeat back to a normal rate.

Tracey's Tips for the Stationary Bike

• Adjust your seat to a comfortable height so that you can push down on the pedal. Your must be able to almost straighten the knee on the downward motion, and the knee should have a 45-degree bend on the upward pedaling motion. The hip, knee, and ankle should be aligned.

• If you're placing your feet in the cages, the straps must be tight and not hanging loose.

• If your foot becomes loose, stop your workout and tighten the straps before cycling again. Otherwise, you could get injured.

• Make sure that your hands are holding on to the handlebars gently (not clinging to them for dear life) and that there is no weight from your torso in your hands. This keeps all the work in your legs!

• Slightly extend the spine and sit upright with the abs contracted at *all* times. If you have any back problems, you may want to try the recumbent bike for support.

• Try going with the beat of the music; this can help keep your pace consistent. Also, watch your RPM gauge for visual feedback.

STATIONARY BIKE

SIX-MINUTE WORKOUT: STATIONARY BIKE

0.00–2.00	LEVEL 0: WARM-UP	RPE 5
2.00–4.00	LEVEL 1: INCREASE PACE	RPE 5.5–6
4.00–5.00	LEVEL 2: INTERVAL INCREASING PACE	RPE 6–7
5.00–5.30	LEVEL 0: DECREASE PACE	RPE 5
5.30–6.00	LEVEL 0: RECOVER	RPE 3–4

THIRTY-MINUTE WORKOUT: STATIONARY BIKE

0.00–5.00	LEVEL 0: WARM-UP	RPE 5
5.00–6.00	LEVEL 1: INCREASE PACE	RPE 5.5–6
6.00–8.00	LEVEL 0: RECOVER	RPE 5
8.00–9.00	LEVEL 1: INCREASE PACE	RPE 5.5–6
9.00–11.00	LEVEL 0: RECOVER	RPE 5
11:00–12.00	LEVEL 2: INCREASE PACE	RPE 6.5–7.5
12.00–15.00	LEVEL 0: RECOVER	RPE 5.5
15.00–16:00	LEVEL 1: INCREASE PACE	RPE 6–7
16:00–19.00	LEVEL 0: RECOVER	RPE 5.5
19.00–22.00	LEVEL 2: INCREASE PACE	RPE 6.5–7.5
22.00–25.00	LEVEL 0: RECOVER	RPE 5.5
25.00–28.00	LEVEL 1: INCREASE PACE	RPE 6–7
28.00–30.00	LEVEL 0: RECOVER AND START TO COOL DOWN	RPE 3.5–5

Start to slow your pedal strokes and take deep breaths to bring your heart rate back down to normal.
At the end of the last two minutes, come to a complete stop.

Tracey's Tip

Hold on to the handlebars and start pedaling. On every stroke, try to imagine that you're pulling up with the heel, activating the hamstrings and glutes. Your feet should always be flexed and your abs pulled in tight, supporting the torso. Take deep breaths as you start to feel your heart rate elevate.

WHO KNEW?

Researchers at the University of Victoria in British Columbia found that dog owners walked an average of three hundred minutes per week compared to just one hundred sixty-eight minutes for those who were Fido-free.

QUICK CARDIO STRETCHES

FIVE ESSENTIAL STRETCHES

Don't forget that you always need to stretch after our cardio sessions. I know it's tempting to move quickly onto the next chore of the day. But don't. Instead, stop and think for one minute what those poor muscles have carried you through. Hills, fast sprints, stairs, a long bike ride. Don't you think they deserve a little pampering? Plus, stretching feels so good not only while you do it, but the next day when your body doesn't feel tight. Do you want to be one of those people who have never stretched a day in their life and can't even lift their legs onto the curb? I know people who wonder why their joints are hurting and why they keep getting injured. To prevent injuries, muscles need regular stretching—we do this by releasing and lengthening, which keeps the muscles supple and loose. If they're too tight, muscles cannot work properly to support the joints.

1. Lunge into Hamstring Stretch

Muscles stretched: Hamstrings and hip flexors

Hold: Thirty seconds in each position

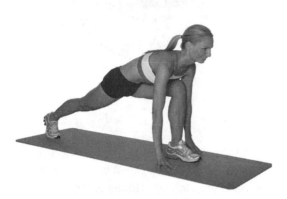 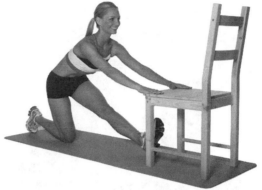

A. Stand in a lunge position with your front leg bent and your hands on either side of your knees, shoulder-width apart. Straighten the back leg and curl your toes under, making sure your hips and thighs are parallel to the floor. Draw in the abdominals so that you do not overarch your back. You will feel the stretch in front of your hips (hip flexors). Hold this stretch for at least thirty seconds.

B. Drop the back knee down to the floor (you may need some cushions if this causes discomfort) and lift the hips back, extending the front leg and resting your foot on your heel. Depending on your flexibility, move your hands back toward your body. Hold for a further thirty seconds.

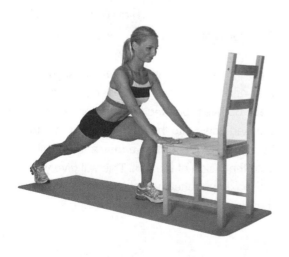

> ### Tracey's Tip
>
> By drawing in, your abs pull your pelvis into a more natural position, resulting in a better hip flexor stretch.

Modification: Hold on to the corners of a chair for support.

2. Figure-Four Hip Stretch

Muscles stretched: Glutes and inner thighs

Hold: Thirty seconds each side

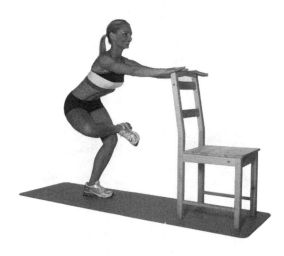

Tracey's Tip

For an extra hip opener, place a little extra weight on your bent knee with your hand.

A. Holding onto a chair or wall for support, cross your right leg on top of your left thigh and bend your left leg. Gently press your hips back as if you were going to sit down. You will feel a stretch in the right hip and glute.

3. Calf Stretch

Muscles stretched: Calves

Hold: Thirty seconds

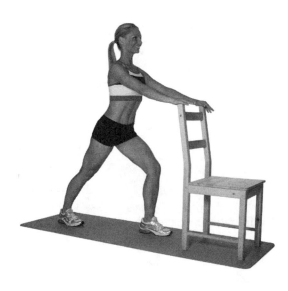

Tracey's Tip

To increase the stretch, slightly pitch your body forward in a diagonal line from the crown of the head to the heel.

A. Holding on to a chair or wall for support, stand tall with your left leg slightly bent and your right leg extended behind you. Keep both feet pointed forward and heels pressed down into the floor. It's important to keep the weight on all five toes and not roll onto the inside of the foot. This will give you the maximum effective stretch for your calf muscles.

4. Quad Stretch

Muscles stretched: Quads

Hold: Thirty to sixty seconds each side

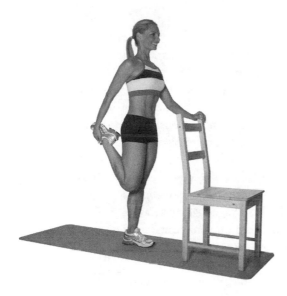

A. Hold onto a chair or wall for support and bend your right leg toward your butt. Hold your right foot with both knees together, drawing the heel toward the butt. Face your hips forward and contract your abs, holding your pelvis still for a greater stretch.

5. Towel Chest and Shoulder Stretch

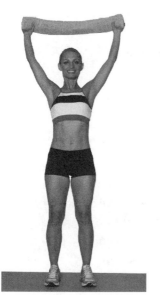

Muscles targeted: Pectorals and shoulders

Reps: 5

You need: Rolled-up towel

A. Stand tall and hold a rolled-up towel in front of your body with your hands shoulder-width apart.

B. Exhale and lift your arms up and over your head until you feel a stretch in your chest and shoulders. Hold for a few seconds, and then return your arms to the starting position and repeat.

**TRACEY'S TOP TEN WAYS TO
SHAKE UP YOUR CARDIO WORKOUT**

1. Work out with a friend.

2. Listen to music.

3. Change your route—it challenges the body. Add hills to work the legs.

4. Sign up for a charity 5K race. You'll get fit while you fund raise and have fun. Find one in your area at www.active.com.

5. Take a new class. Whether it's dance, kick boxing, or spinning, trying something different is fun.

6. Try active recreational activities such as hiking with your husband, friends, or kids or outdoor bike riding. It's so much fun you won't realize that you're burning calories.

7. Download workouts from Web sites such as iamplify.com. You get fun new workouts and have your own personal trainer. (I'm one of them.)

8. Add small intervals to your daily run, walk, bike, or elliptical routine.

9. Get a pedometer (a little device you hang on your pants and use to count the steps you take). You'll find that you'll start challenging yourself.

10. Hire a personal trainer for just one or two sessions (or split them with a friend). You'll learn some new workouts and get invaluable tips on form.

IF YOU'RE TIGHT ON TIME, WALK THIS WAY!

Most of us take about 3,000 steps per day, but to burn calories and slim down, you need to get closer to 10,000 steps per day, which is equal to about 5 miles. Don't worry, you don't have to count every step. Just get a pedometer and it'll do that for you.

Research from the University of Minnesota found that pedometers get people on their feet and strolling away. Wearing it all day gives you a sense of how many steps you currently take, and there's something about having one on that makes you walk a little more. And a pedometer is a great option if you just can't find the time for any bonus cardio. Go talk to that coworker instead of sending an e-mail, or bring the laundry to your child's room instead of waiting for him or her to come get it. I know that when I wear one I get into a little competition with myself. Can I step more today than yesterday? Should I park a little farther from the grocery store so I get a few more steps in? Should I get the paper instead of waiting for my husband? Trust me, it's surprisingly easy and kind of fun! You don't have to spend a ton of money on this gadget. They come in all price ranges but those at the lower end—around $20—work just fine.

To start, I recommend that you simply wear your pedometer for three days and record the number of steps that you naturally take. Then figure out your average and gradually increase this by twenty percent every week. Better yet, have a competition with your partner or best friend and see who can take the most steps each week. A little competition never hurt anyone!

WHO KNEW?

Cleaning house counts as cardio! On the average, you burn 150 calories per hour vacuuming, dusting, mopping, or washing windows.

CALORIE EXPENDITURES

Here's an estimate of how many calories you torch doing thirty minutes of various cardio workouts. The following numbers are based on people with about 20 percent body fat:

- Aerobics (low impact): 185 calories
- 10-mph cycling (moderate): 300 calories
- 15-mph cycling (vigorous): 480 calories
- Swimming: 265 calories
- Walking (moderate): 145 calories
- Walking (vigorous): 195 calories

WHO KNEW?

According to the Centers for Disease Control and Prevention (CDC), obesity rates have nearly doubled from an estimated 15 percent in 1980 to nearly 27 percent today!

COMMON CARDIO INJURIES

Plantar Fasciitis

Usual symptom: Pain in the arches of the feet.

Causes: Overpronation of the feet (a fancy way of saying that the arches are rolling in), tight calves, and unsupportive running shoes.

Prevention: Gently massage the arches of the feet to loosen up tight muscles, and invest in a pair of running shoes with good arch support.

Try this: Place a tennis ball under the arches of your feet and gently roll it back and forth, adding more pressure as the muscles start to release tension.

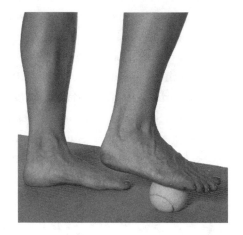

Achilles Tendonitis

Usual symptom: Pain in the heel where the tendon attaches at the heel.

Causes: Tight calf muscles over time will pull on the Achilles tendon and create strain, causing inflammation and pain.

Prevention: Stretch the calves before and after doing any kind of exercise, especially running.

Try this: Holding on to a wall for support, step the right leg behind the left and bend your left knee. Press your right heel into the floor with the toes pointing forward and slightly pitch your body forward with your abs pulled in. Feel the stretch in the calf and hold for at least thirty seconds to one minute. Switch legs and repeat.

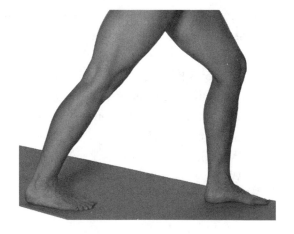

PAIN IN YOUR KNEES

Wondering why your knees ache? Pain in the lateral part (sides) of the knee is a common complaint from runners and bikers. Both of these workouts cause tightness of the quadriceps, glutes, and tensor fascia lata, or TFL, the long muscle that runs from the hip and down the thigh and attaches at the knee. Quad tightness causes increased pressure on the patella (the kneecap) and leads to pain underneath it due to the compression. TFL and glute tightness causes tightening of the iliotibial, or IT, band and leads to a lateral (sideway) pull of the patella (misalignment). This can also cause pain in the knee due to the patella being pulled out of its natural alignment. The repetitive action of running and biking only makes these problems worse.

Try this: Gentle stretching and self-massage releases tension of these muscles and stops them pulling on the kneecap, preventing knee pain.

Self-Massage of the IT Band with Foam Roller

To self-massage the IT band, I like to use body-rolling balls or foam rollers. (Appendix C lists places where you can purchase them.)

Purpose: To give yourself a self-massage and loosen the IT band.

A. Lie sideways with your hip on the foam roller and both hands on the floor in front of your body. (This controls how much pressure will go on the ball.) Start at the hip and roll the foam roller down the side of leg. You'll know when you've found the right muscle because you will feel tenderness.

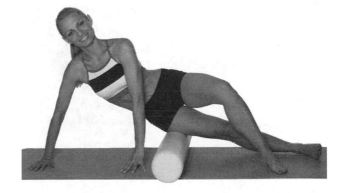

B. Hold for thirty seconds, and then continue up the leg. Switch sides and repeat. Do this every day before and after you run or bike.

IT Band Stretch

Purpose: To stretch out the hamstring and IT band.

A. Lie on your back with your right leg extended and supported with a Theraband (exercise band) or a large rolled-up towel hooked around the instep of your foot.

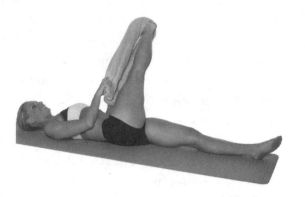

B. Pull your leg gently toward you and then internally rotate the leg and toe so that they're facing toward your left shoulder. Slightly cross the leg toward your left shoulder, feeling the stretch down the side of the leg and calf muscles. Switch legs and repeat. Do this stretch two times before and after running. Hold for at least thirty seconds.

Success Story

Michelle Eaton, 37, Seattle, Washington

Lost

11 pounds
4 percent body fat
Two dress sizes
1 inch of her arms
4 inches of her waist
3 inches of her hips
1 inch of her thighs
9 inches total

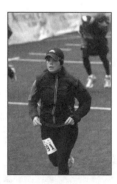

Before

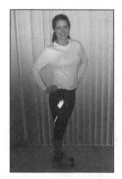

After

Gained

Stronger abs and no more lower back pain, *something I've suffered with for many years. This allowed me to run farther without discomfort.*

• • • • •

Over the years, Michelle Eaton's weight fluctuated 15 pounds up and down. "The extra weight made me feel sluggish and chubby and like I had little personal discipline," says this 37-year-old office manager. Although Michelle ran half marathons and marathons, she wasn't as fit as she wanted to be. "I didn't consider myself healthy or in shape," she says. Boredom had also set into her exercise life and she longed to feel excited about working out again.

The answer to her fitness prayers was Tracey's DVD. "It makes you feel as if Tracey is working out with you and helping you reach your potential and the next level of fitness," she says. "I loved that the workouts had a lot of variety so it wasn't the same thing every day." Tracey also helped spice up Michelle's passion for running. Instead of her normal forty-five to fifty minutes running, she tried the interval workouts Tracey created and was amazed at how quickly the time passed and how much she enjoyed the treadmill. "This is important in Seattle, where it often pours and you can't always run outside," she says.

Food had also been another challenge in Michelle's life. In the past, she'd tried programs that taught her portion control but didn't offer enough flexibility or options for her vegetarian diet. At first, it was tough to adjust to eating the five to six small meals a day and the amount of pro-

MICHELLE'S STICK-WITH-IT TIP

Follow the meal plan closely. Eating six small meals a day curbed any tendencies to binge or overeat at one particular meal. And, surprisingly, my sugar cravings were satisfied by the high protein and naturally sweet foods. Before the program, I was eating the wrong foods at the wrong times, and during the middle of a run or a video tape, I would experience tiredness and stomach cramps from lack of energy. On Tracey's food plan, my energy level increased in just the first few weeks.

tein that Tracey recommends, but with time she understood why this method was so effective. "Eating the right blend of foods didn't make me feel deprived," says Michelle. "Unlike other diets I've been on, I never felt starved or unsatisfied. My tendency to overeat slowly went away and I learned to make wiser choices. And when I did indulge in higher fat foods, I enjoyed them without the need to pig out." Plus, the meal plan gave Michelle the energy boost she needed to get through her evening workouts without hunger pains. "I really can push through a set even when I am tired," she says.

What she liked most about *Sexy in 6* was being able to easily tailor it to it her life. "You can make the changes that work for you and your goals and lifestyle," she says. "The program provides a lot of variety and you're able to pick and choose exercises, food, and goals that work just for you." Plus, the chronic low-back pain Michelle suffered thanks to running decreased by the end of the six weeks. "My back muscles were my weakest, but they're so much stronger after doing the program." As a result, Michelle stands up taller—literally and figuratively. "Today, my clothes fit better instead of being snug. But more importantly," she says, "my posture is improved and I carry my body with so much more confidence."

TRACEY'S TAKE

Michelle is a typical example that doing cardio alone and not watching food portions will not get results! Although she was in good cardiovascular shape, the same old workout every day was ruining her motivation. Strength training and intervals were exactly what Michelle needed to boost her metabolism and swap fat for lean muscle. Michelle has signed up for her next marathon in October and I *know* she'll make it to that finish line!

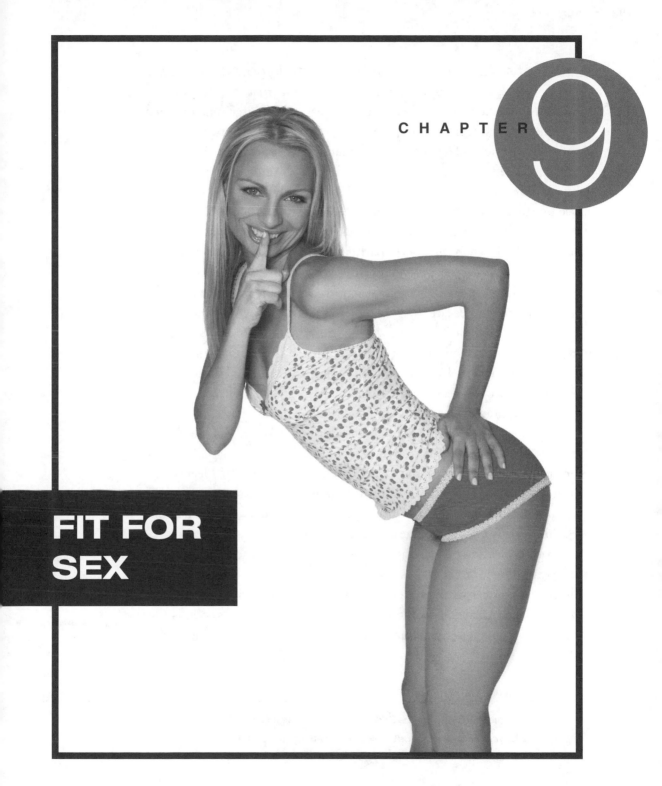

CHAPTER 9

FIT FOR
SEX

ET'S TALK ABOUT SEX, BABY. YES, SEX. I KNOW IT MAY *SEEM* like a strange topic in a fitness book, but trust me, the two are connected. In fact, exercise is the secret to better sex, stronger orgasms, and longer staying power. "Being in better shape improves your sex life for a few reasons," explains Ava Cadell, Ph.D., a Los Angeles–based sex therapist, author of eight books including *12 Steps to Everlasting Love,* and founder of the Loveology University. First, exercise increases blood circulation throughout your entire body. And when I say your *entire* body I mean it—so down there gets a boost in blood flow, too. Well when *that* body part gets more blood flow, it increases your sensitivity, arousal, and chance of having an orgasm. So exercising not only slims you down but can rev up your sex life too. Running for your workout clothes already? Wait, there's more.

Studies show that the more weight you lose, the more your sex life improves: A Duke University study found that even a 10 percent reduction in weight (that's 15 pounds if you weigh 150) resulted in major improvements in all areas of the participant's sex life, such as arousal, feelings of attractiveness, and enjoyment of sexual activity. If you look good, you're going to feel better about your body. And if you feel better about your body, chances are you're going to feel sexier, right? (Works for me every time!) One of the Team Mallett members said, "I feel sexier in my new body and I don't want to hide under the covers anymore." She not only has more energy for sex, but her stronger and more flexible legs are great for being more creative. You go girl!

Experts also say that having sex and an orgasm releases the hormone oxytocin. This in turn causes the release of the same feel-good endorphins that you get when you eat chocolate or exercise. Sex is similar to exercise also because it's another great way to relieve stress. Sex is the time to completely let go, enjoy the moment, and stop thinking about

MOTIVATION FROM TEAM MALLETT

It's easier to be more confident in the bedroom when your significant other is so impressed with your progress that he's paying more attention. I also find I want to be touched and massaged more now that my bulges are turning into curves.
—Anonymous

your to-do list. There are even studies showing that sex lowers your blood pressure for up to a week.

Here's another way sex and exercise are linked: There are ways you can tone up down below so that your time spent under the covers is even more satisfying. The pelvic floor area is usually the weakest and most neglected area in the entire body, but these muscles are the most important for heightened sexual pleasure for both partners. If you've had a baby and delivered vaginally, these muscles are usually weak and stretched out. "Pelvic floor muscle strengthening exercises have been shown to overcome some of the adverse effects of vaginal delivery and other causes of pelvic floor muscle relaxation," says Howard Kaufman, M.D., associate professor of Surgery and Obstetrics and Gynecology at the Keck School of Medicine at the University of Southern California (USC). The exercises Dr. Kaufman is referring to are kegels (something we discussed in chapter 6). I swear that they're the secret for hotter sex and intense orgasms. (That Team Mallett member I mentioned e-mailed me around week four to tell me about the "atomic orgasm" she'd had the night before. Not exactly the kind of info I expected on her weekly progress reports, but we should all be so lucky!)

One of the many functions of the pelvic floor muscles is to facilitate uterine contractions during childbirth and during an orgasm. Stimulating the nerve endings through regular contraction of the pelvic floor (by doing kegels) ensures a healthy blood flow to this area. Your partner might think that you feel tighter down there as your muscles become more toned. After all, the pelvic floor muscles are the same as any other muscle in your body. A little work and they become more fit. "Core strengthening with Pilates also helps to coordinate the other deep stabilizing muscles of the torso with the pelvic floor muscles," adds Dr. Kaufman.

I should also mention that the *more* orgasms you have, the stronger the pelvic floor gets. A win-win situation for everyone!

"Research shows that the act of sexual intercourse burns about 200 calories, which is equal to running on a treadmill for half an hour," adds Dr. Cadell. "Sex is really an integral part of a healthy life and can help

WHO KNEW?

Stop smoking! And have your partner quit, too. Besides all the health risks, smoking adds wrinkles and makes your teeth yellow, so you won't feel very sexy. Plus, it has a negative effect on your circulation, which means less blood flow throughout the body, including your privates!

you emotionally, psychologically, and physically. It is good for your cardiovascular system, your respiratory system, and menstrual cramps, acts as a laxative, keeps your organs healthy, acts as an antidepressant and a mild sedative, and can stimulate creativity and concentration." Now *I'm* running for my workout gear.

SOLO SEXERCISES

You can get fit for sex when your partner is not around with a few quick and easy moves. Do these exercises at least a few times a week. You should also be doing at least 50 kegel contractions a day just for maintenance. Remember that you can do kegels anywhere—while sitting in your car, in line at Starbucks, or in a meeting. (I promise that I won't tell.)

WHO KNEW?

Stress can squash your libido and thus your sex life. That's just another reason to try yoga or meditation or at the very least take the time each day for a few quiet moments and deep breaths. This time is for focusing on just you, no one else. This has helped me reduce my stress level—and I'm a classic type A personality.

MOTIVATION FROM TEAM MALLETT

My husband says I am hot all the time; he even brags to his coworkers about how in shape I am.
—*Dana Davy-Bench, 27, Elk Grove, California*

1. Pillow Squeezes with Pelvic Tilts

Inspiration: Intense orgasms!

Targets: The pelvic floor, inner thighs, and abs

Tracey's Tip

Try not to use the glutes or hip flexors as you tilt the pelvis. The abs should be doing all the work.

A. Lie on your back with your hands by the sides of your body. Bend your knees and place your feet on the floor with your heels in line with your sit bones. Place a pillow between your thighs and squeeze your legs to hold the pillow in place.

B. Exhale and draw your abs toward the spine as you contract your pelvic floor. Lead with your pubic bone and flatten the lower spine as you tilt your pelvis forward. Inhale and return the pelvis back to a neutral position.

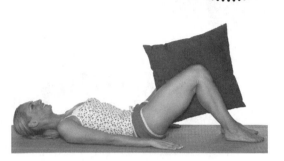

2. Heel Clicks

Inspiration: Stronger leg grip

Muscles targeted: Inner thighs, glutes, and pelvic floor

Reps: 20–40, until you're tired

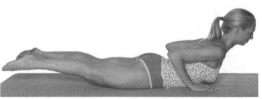

A. Lie on your front with your elbows bent and your hands resting on the floor by your rib cage. Lift your chest off the floor and extend the upper spine. Draw your shoulder blades down your back and straighten your legs, turning them out at the hips with your feet in a small V position and toes pointed.

B. Press your pubic bone into the mat, lifting your legs slightly off the floor. Open your legs hip-width apart and close them quickly, drawing the inner thighs and heels together. Repeat this motion 20–40 times, and then lower your legs and upper body.

Tracey's Tip

Keep your knees off the floor and your hips turned out at all times and think of pressing your pubic bone into the floor so you're extending at the hip.

3. Elevated Pelvic Thrusts

Inspiration: Longer staying power without those nagging cramps in the legs.

Muscles targeted: Glutes, hamstrings, and pelvic floor

Reps: 10–15

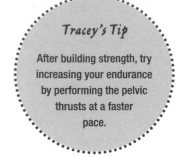

Tracey's Tip

After building strength, try increasing your endurance by performing the pelvic thrusts at a faster pace.

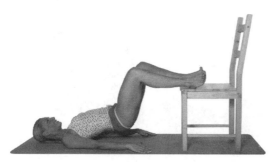

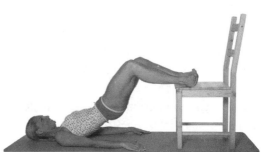

A. Lie on your back with your legs propped up on a chair, hip-width apart. Turn your legs out at the hips with your knees bent. Point your toes out to the corners of the room. Lift your hips off the floor, maintaining a neutral spine.

B. Exhale and contract the abs, drawing your pelvic floor up and tilting your pubic bone up toward the ceiling. Inhale and return to a neutral spine without lowering the hips. Repeat 10–15 times before lowering your butt down to the floor. Finish in the starting position.

4. Happy Baby Pose

Inspiration: The crazy, fun positions you can do with your mate (and keep boredom away)!

Muscles targeted: Inner thighs, lower back, hamstrings, and glutes

Hold: 30–60 seconds

Tracey's Tip

Draw your abs toward the spine and lift your tailbone off the floor about an inch. You will feel a stretch through the hips and the inner thighs.

A. Lie on your back with your legs bent comfortably out to the sides of your body. Wrap your hands around your flexed feet, holding onto the outside of the feet and arches.

B. Draw your feet slightly toward your body to a place that feels comfortable and point your knees out to the corners of the room.

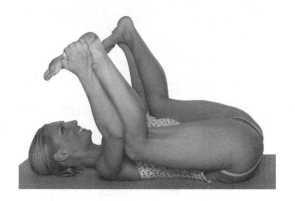

PARTNER SEXERCISES

Here are some exercises you can practice while you're having sex. I'm sure your mate won't mind when you say it's time to work out. And this will be one sweat session you'll never lose motivation for. I call them the sit exercises (which coincidentally is the position you need to be in during this fun workout). There are three exercises, and you should do them in the order shown, with a few minutes of rest in between. (Sorry, no photos for these moves because my husband's a little camera shy, and in this case, so am I!) Sit or squat on top of your partner for all three exercises. You will be amazed how different sex will feel for both of you from doing these three little moves.

1. The Squeeze

A. Sit or squat on top of your partner, allowing deep penetration, and grip the penis as tight as you can with the pelvic floor muscles (again, you do this by acting as if you're trying to stop the flow of urine while peeing). Do this without contracting the glutes, thighs, and abs; the only muscles working should be your pelvic floor muscles.

B. Hold for about twenty seconds, pause ten seconds, and repeat until your partner feels the strength of the contractions decrease.

2. The Insert

A. Slowly insert the penis into the vagina and start contracting the pelvic floor muscles around the penis. You should feel the pelvic floor lift like an elevator.

B. Hold this contraction for ten seconds and slowly release. Repeat five times.

3. The Thrust

Now that you have those pelvic floor muscles in gear (and your guy is totally going nuts!), you're ready for the thrust technique. Try integrating the previous two exercises together with faster-paced pelvic tilts controlled by either you or your partner. Don't forget to stimulate the entire pelvic floor muscles; the sides sometimes get left out!

TIPS FROM THE PROS: HAVE MORE SEX!

Besides the fun factor, here Dr. Ava gives several other reasons why regular sex is a good idea.

• Sex may ward off pesky colds and the flu. Researchers at Wilkes University in Pennsylvania discovered that people who had regular sex had 30 percent higher levels of immunoglobulin A, an antibody that boosts the immune system.

• Sex boosts blood flow to all your organs, which keeps everything in good working condition from top to bottom.

• Sex can be an effective antidepressant because it causes the brain to release a feel-good neurotransmitter called dopamine.

• The physical and emotional aspects of sex can work together to improve self-esteem and self-confidence.

• Sex can help get your creative juices flowing. Because sexual fulfillment also involves your brain, it can improve a variety of mental functions, including your concentration.

• Sex benefits neck and back muscles, which increases blood flow to the brain and can alleviate certain types of headache. So, the next time your partner says, "I have a headache" you can say, "Good, let's make love and get rid of it."

Success Story

....

*Robin Wood, 48, married, mother of one, accountant,
Fayetteville, North Carolina*

Lost

11 pounds

8 percent body fat

Three dress sizes

3 inches off her chest

4 inches off her waist

2 ½ inches off her hips

9 ½ inches total

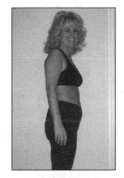

Before

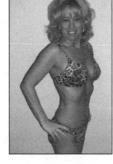

After

Gained

Freedom from hot flashes. *After my hysterectomy I started having meno-
pausal symptoms, but I haven't had any since I started Tracey's program—
not a single hot flash and no night sweats.*

• • • • •

Most of her adult life, Robin Wood's weight fluctuated up or down 15
pounds. In her 40s, it stayed on the upper end of that spectrum and she
found it harder and harder to slim down. "I was overweight and flabby. I
didn't like how I looked in clothes and I definitely didn't like what I saw
out of my clothes," she says. "I was very self-conscious about my appearance and hated going out because I had to struggle to find something to

ROBIN'S STICK-WITH-IT TIP

*Dedicate yourself to two weeks. Commit yourself to a finite number of weeks and the
program will become part of your life. You'll enjoy the results so much you won't want
to stop. You should feel good knowing that this program has been tried by a variety of
people and has been proven to be successful. I committed to this program because it
promised results and I trusted that Tracey could deliver on her promise. She did!*

wear." Robin was also bothered by her lower ab bulge, a problem spot that only got worse after she had a hysterectomy.

"When I first saw Tracey's workouts I was a little intimidated by the six-day-a-week schedule. I thought I would never be able to do that much," says Robin. All that changed after just one week. "The more I exercised, the more I *wanted* to exercise. Now it's such a part of my daily routine that I don't want to miss a day," says Robin, who loved the small six-minute segments that she could "mix and match." "Now that I've learned what it takes to get the results that I want, I no longer feel like working out is a constant battle. Now it's my ally and I'm motivated to do it every time I look in the mirror." The other reward she reaped for her hard work? Her problem spot is far from a problem. "I do my abdominal exercises every day now that I know that twelve minutes a day is all it takes to have amazing abs," she says. "Just twelve minutes!"

Robin's pre-Tracey diet included a lot of pizza, hero sandwiches, hamburgers, and fries, and snacking on chips, crackers, and cheese before and after dinner. Another no-no: she picked at uneaten food on her husband and son's plates. On Tracey's plan, Robin found satisfying, healthy snacks she enjoyed and paid attention to portion size. "Also, the idea of eating a little before going out to dinner was great advice because social events are unavoidable," she says. Amazingly, Robin says making all these changes in her life was pretty easy. "I know it doesn't seem possible, but I really didn't find anything particularly hard. I just followed the program and my body shaped itself."

Gone is the old Robin who liked to stay at home, didn't care about her appearance, and hated shopping. After six weeks, she went shopping for capri pants and brought a size 7 into the dressing room only to find

MOTIVATION FROM TEAM MALLETT

This may be too much information, but an unexpected result of daily exercise is an increase in sexual desire. I have so much more energy that sex is becoming an outlet for it. Also, with increased flexibility and the strength to hold various positions longer there is a whole new world of mobility and acrobatics opening up! Lastly, an increase in self-confidence makes me more apt to try new things. Because I no longer worry how much my belly hangs out, I focus my attention on, well, other matters!
—*Tanya Torforson, 28, Bruderheim, Canada*

that it was too big. The same thing happened again and again, and she wound up buying a size 1! "I remember how depressing it was to try on clothes when I was heavy," she recalls. "Now, everything I try on looks great and that can get very expensive." But it's all worth it for a figure she never knew was possible. Another unpredictable bonus? "The plan definitely improved my sex life! My increased energy level affected the frequency of sex and my flexibility and stamina made it more creative. Plus, I felt sexier with my new shapely body," she says. "I'm so amazed that at age 48, I look the best I ever have. I feel empowered now that I know the secret to having a great body."

TRACEY'S TAKE

Robin is hot, hot, hot! When I saw her final picture I nearly fell off my chair—I was so amazed at how fabulous she looked. Her biggest goal starting this program was to finally get rid of the 40s hormonal tummy pooch. Robin learned that quality is far superior to quantity and overall conditioning is the key. No matter how hard you try, you can't spot-reduce. Robin is definitely *Sexy in 6* with a load of newfound confidence. All I can say is that her husband had better watch out!

MOTIVATION FROM TEAM MALLETT

This program is really helping my relationship with my husband because he sees me making an effort.
—Randi Hsu, 42, Short Hills, New Jersey

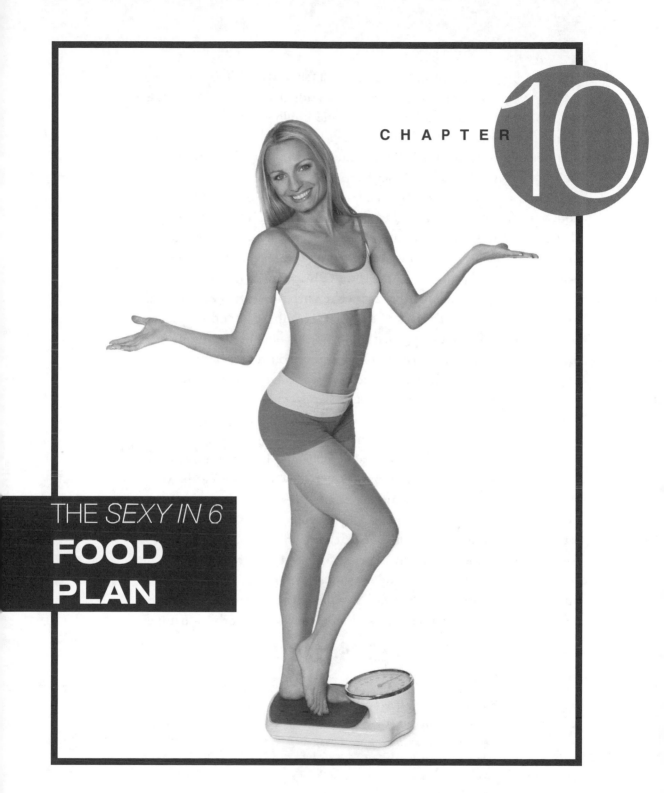

CHAPTER 10

THE *SEXY IN 6*
**FOOD
PLAN**

M Y PROGRAM INCLUDES A HEALTHY EATING PLAN. IT'S THE plan I used to shed the 55 pounds that I packed on while pregnant, and it's the same one I follow today. It's how my clients trim down and how Team Mallett lost a total of more than 400 pounds. Yes, 400 pounds! They went nuts for this eating plan and couldn't believe how satisfied they were.

This is a plan, not a *diet*. Say the D-word and most of us think starvation, a growling stomach, and eating naked lettuce. This is a lifestyle change. It's a healthy way of eating that you can use forever, not just for the next six weeks. It lets you indulge but also teaches you how to control portions. And portions are the key. I've heard many nutritionists say that if people just ate less of what they're currently eating they'd lose weight. Imagine that! Eat less of that pizza, hamburger, and ice cream and slim down. I'm not saying that those foods should be staples in your diet, but my point is that the effect of portion size on your weight is huge. Obviously, to lose weight you need to eat fewer calories. However, when you're eventually at a weight that you're happy with, there's still no excuse to binge on fast food and desserts. The classic line "everything in moderation" is the perfect way to summarize eating.

I've tried my best to make this eating plan a no-brainer (hey, I know you're busy) by listing the foods and exactly how much you're allowed. What I love is that we're not counting calories; it's all about portion control. After all, when you're starving, tallying your calories with a calculator just isn't going to happen. But by eating smaller portions, you're naturally controlling how many calories you eat—no math required!

I've also made sure that many of the foods in my plan work double-duty to slim you down while giving you the nutrients you need to ward off disease, enhance your energy, and look your best. Food is a natural

MOTIVATION FROM TEAM MALLETT

The biggest surprise was finding healthy,
convenient ways to have good meals and snacks.
I love food and love eating and this plan makes it easy.
—Alison Fukomoto, 29, Santa Monica, California

medicine, and researchers are learning more about its benefits almost daily. One example is veggies. They're filled with disease-fighting anti-oxidants (another reason why half your plate should be brimming with these goodies-from-the-garden). I believe that the old saying "You are what you eat" is true. Do you want to look dull and bumpy like a piece of batter-fried chicken or bright, smooth, and sleek like a piece of salmon?

Tracey's Tip

Women who see a big change in the first two weeks are more likely to keep with the plan, so be firm with yourself!

In the next chapter, I talk in detail about how you can use common objects to eyeball the right quantities of food. This takes practice, so for the first week or two, pull out those measuring cups and spoons and a scale and measure your food. At first, what you see will surprise you.

Many members of Team Mallett were stunned when they saw what correct portion sizes actually looked like. In fact, I had a few skeptics in the bunch who were adamant that their diets weren't preventing them from slimming down. According to them, they were eating the right foods and the proper amounts. Sure, some were, but some were way off. And I don't blame them. We get accustomed to gargantuan-size portions, so when we see a correct portion we think it's a meal made for a mouse. I'm giving you the tools to regain control over what goes into your body. This program will teach you to make better choices and understand portion sizes. When you have these two simple facts embedded in your brain, you're set for life! Let's get going.

HOW DOES THE HEALTHY EATING PLAN WORK?

You're allowed the following portions every day:

Seven protein
Three dairy
Four fruit
Five grain
Three fat
Unlimited veggies
Unlimited glasses of water

In the beginning, I suggest skipping alcohol because it's empty calories that can add up. I love a nice glass of wine just like the next gal, but it's best to hold off when you're trying to shed pounds. For those who cannot do without alcohol, limit it to no more than four alcoholic drinks a week.

THE SUPER-EASY FOOD LOG

Yes, I know lots of women hate keeping a food log, but trust me, it works. Studies have found it to be effective, and it's the only way you can be honest with yourself.

Human nature helps us forget the things we don't want to remember, such as the pizza crust you ate from your kid's plate or the doughnut no one saw you chow down at the office. One client of mine was frustrated because she couldn't seem to lose weight. Finally, I told her to write down everything she ate. She did this for a week and was stunned at all the nibbles and noshes she consumed throughout the day. Just a pizza crust, a cookie, and a few stray fries each day can add up to more than 200 calories. Do that daily and by the end of the week that's 1,000 calories! Over a month that's 4,000 calories. Eating 3,500 calories makes you gain a pound, so you can do the math and see how mindless eating is a problem. When you have to write down what you eat, you think twice about putting just anything in your mouth. Always be honest with yourself; the only person you're letting down is you.

The good news is that I've made the food log easy for you. First, photocopy the sample page I have in Appendix A so you have a sheet for every day (or you can download it from my website, www.traceymallett.com). The second reason why it's a cinch? You don't have to write down lengthy descriptions of what you ate. In fact, you don't have to write much. Here's how it works: Each food you eat will correspond to one of the food portions in the

Sweets—they are everywhere and easy to "accidentally" eat. But writing down what I ate for a few weeks showed me that I was eating fewer fruits and vegetables than I should. Now I really go out of my way to eat more of both. I love to use my rice cooker to steam vegetables a bunch at a time—the flavor is amazing and it's so fast and easy.
—Erin Lamb, 37, San Marino, California

different food columns. For example, if you eat a ½ cup of rice, you cross out a G for grains. If you eat an egg, cross out a D for dairy. All the columns should always add up to the amounts in the total column. All the portions amounts are explained on page 208.

I also recommend that you write down the following valuable information. This will help you identify stressful situations, foods that make you more satisfied, and the times of day when you need to be prepared with healthy treats.

Each log should include the following.

1. The times you ate.
2. The times you were the hungriest.
3. Stressful situations (why you overate, such as you were bored, lonely, or had problems)
4. How you felt after overeating.
5. All positive thoughts!

After a few days, you will start to see a pattern of your eating habits and stressful triggers to try to avoid.

Following is a sample of how to use your daily food journal.

EXAMPLE—TEAM MALLETT FOOD LOG

	Protein	Dairy	Grains	Fruits	Fats	Veggies (nonstarches)	Water
Breakfast	P P P P	D D	G G	F	FATS	V V V	W W
Snack	P P	D D	G	F F		V V V	W
Lunch	P P P P	D D	G G	F	FATS	V V V	W W
Snack	P P	D D	G	F F		V V V	W
Dinner	P P P P	D D	G G	F	FATS	V V V	W W
Evening snack (optional)	P P	D D	G	F F	FATS	V V V	W
Day's Maximum	7	3	5	4	3	Unlimited	Unlimited
DAY'S TOTAL	7	3	5	4	3	8	8

Journal Your Treat: One glass of red wine 4oz

Daily Notes: Feeling good today. I was told by my co-worker that I looked smaller.

Ate breakfast at 6am. Snack at 9am. Lunch at 12pm. Afternoon snack at 3pm. Dinner at 6pm. No evening snack today.

FOOD PLAN

PROTEIN

Servings per day: Seven

Note: Some protein entries include + *one fat*. These foods have a higher fat content so they count as one protein and one fat on your food planner.

Poultry
1 ounce chicken or turkey, without skin
1 ounce chicken or turkey, dark meat or with skin, + one fat

Tracey's Tips

- Eat red meat only one to two times a week.
- Stay away from processed, packaged meat; it's high in hidden sugar and sodium. Instead, buy fresh meat at the deli section.
- Don't eat fish more than four times a week due to the mercury levels that may be present.
- Don't depend on cheese for protein or calcium.

Fish
1 ounce catfish
1 ounce haddock
1 ounce mahi mahi
1 ounce salmon
1 ounce sea bass
1 ounce sole
1 ounce canned salmon, packed in water, not oil
1 ounce canned tuna, packed in water, not oil

Shellfish
1 ounce clams
1 ounce crab
1 ounce imitation shellfish
1 ounce lobster
1 ounce scallops
1 ounce shrimp

Beef
1 ounce beef (USDA select or choice grades of lean meat with visible fat trimmed)

Pork
1 ounce lean pork
1 slice bacon, + one fat
1 slice Canadian bacon

Lamb
1 ounce lamb (roast, chop, or leg)

Soy
½ cup tofu
½ cup tempeh
1 soy hot dog

Eggs

1 whole egg

2 egg whites

½ cup egg substitute

Other

1 low-fat turkey, beef, or pork hot dog,
    + one fat

1 tablespoon natural peanut butter,
    almond butter, or nut butter, + one fat

DAIRY

Servings per day: Three

Note: Some dairy entries include + *one fat*. These foods have a higher fat content, so they count as one dairy and one fat on your food planner.

Milk

1 cup fat-free milk

1 cup 2% fat milk, + one fat

1 cup fat-free or low-fat soy milk

1 cup fat-free or low-fat yogurt (my new
    favorite is Dannon Activia, which
    contains healthy bacteria that help keep
    your digestive system in shape)

Cheese

1 ounce reduced-fat cheese:

American

Cheddar

Feta

Goat

Monterey jack

Swiss

½ cup low-fat cottage cheese

1 tablespoon grated parmesan cheese

1 ounce part-skim mozzarella cheese

¼ cup (2 ounces) fat-free or low-fat ricotta

1 ounce soy cheese

MOTIVATION FROM TEAM MALLETT

*I love that the healthy eating plan is easy to prepare for and follow.
It doesn't require specialty products or foods I've never heard of.
It's just wholesome fresh foods and it all makes complete sense!*
—Valerie Horrey-Wold, 41, South Pasadena, California

VEGGIES

Servings per day: Unlimited

Note: Yes, you read that correctly. It's rare to find people who overeat veggies. In fact, most of us eat considerably less than what's required for a healthy daily intake (at least five servings a day). So go on, be a devil and fill up your plate! And when a craving strikes, try eating veggies first. Their fiber and water may fill you up and keep your hand out of the cookie jar. However, starchy veggies such as potatoes, corn, and peas are not included under this category; check the grains.

½ cup cooked or 1 cup raw veggies equals 25 calories

Some Good Options
Recently, I was at a fancy Palm Springs resort and ordered a plate of veggies with *no butter*. When the server came back with the veggies, they were swimming in the stuff. It was more like an order of butter with veggies on the side. My husband was mortified that I wanted to send them back and snapped at me to "Just eat them." No dice! Saving face (his, not mine) was not worth the hundreds of calories. I had a glass of wine instead!

Artichoke	Eggplant
Arugula	Green beans
Artichoke hearts	Green onions
Asparagus	Leeks
Bean sprouts	Mushrooms
Beets	Onions
Broccoli	Peppers
Brussels sprouts	Radishes
Cabbage	Salad greens
Carrots	Spinach
Cauliflower	Tomato
Celery	Turnips
Chilies	Watercress
Cucumber	Zucchini

FRUITS

Servings per day: Four

1 small apple (4 ounces)
½ cup unsweetened applesauce
4 apricots
1 small banana
1 cup blackberries
1 cup blueberries
1 cup cubed cantaloupe
1 cup (3 ounces) fresh cherries
3 dates
Half large grapefruit (11 ounces)
1 cup (3 ounces) grapes
1 cup (10 ounces) cubed honeydew
1 kiwi
1 cup mandarin orange
Half a small mango
1 small nectarine
1 small orange
½ or 1 cup cubed papaya
1 medium peach (4 ounces)
½ large fresh pear (4 ounces)

1 cup cubed fresh pineapple
2 small plums (5 ounces)
3 prunes
2 tablespoons raisins
1 cup raspberries
1¼ cup strawberries
2 small tangerines
1¼ cup cubed watermelon

Unsweetened Fruit Juice
Note: Natural juice, no added sugar.
Whole fruit is a better choice than fruit
juice because it contains more fiber.
Try to consume fruit first!

⅓ cup grape juice
½ cup grapefruit juice
⅓ cup orange juice
⅓ cup pineapple juice
⅓ cup pomegranate juice

MOTIVATION FROM TEAM MALLETT

*The most surprising thing about this program is the food plan. I thought I had a
healthy diet before I started this and didn't want to become so focused on food
because I was worried it would have a damaging affect on my mind and wouldn't
be good for my daughters to see me so focused on the food part. But I followed it
and my whole family has benefited. I found that while I ate healthy foods before
I wasn't getting a very balanced diet. I didn't get nearly enough protein, fruits, or
vegetables and I was surprised to find that keeping my blood sugar balanced
has resulted in fewer dips in energy midday and a real decline in cravings.*
—Liz Price, 37, South Pasadena, California

GRAINS AND STARCHY VEGGIES

Servings per day: Five

Note: Some grain entries include + *one fat*. These foods have a higher fat content, so they count as one grain and one fat on your food planner.

Breads

1 slice of whole grain bread (check that the bread has at least 3 grams of fiber per slice)

2 slices of light bread (50 calories per slice)

½ English muffin

½ 6-inch-round wheat pita bread

½ small hamburger or hot dog bun

1 6-inch-round wheat tortilla

¼ slice of naan bread

1 small plain dinner roll

1 slice plain raisin bread

1 cup whole-wheat baked croutons

4-inch reduced-fat square waffle

Pasta and Grains

½ cup cooked whole grain pasta

½ cup cooked brown rice

½ cup cooked quinoa

½ cup cooked couscous

¼ cup hummus, + one fat

Cereals

½ cup cooked oatmeal (steel-cut is the most nutritious)

½ cup cooked barley

1 cup bran flakes cereal

1 cup oat rings

½ cup bulgur

¼ cup low-fat granola (less than 10g of fat per serving)

½ cup cooked kasha

½ cup cooked millet

½ cup muesli

½ cup or 1 biscuit shredded wheat

1½ bricks Weetabix

Crackers

8 animal crackers

8 small pretzels

3 2½-inch square graham crackers

4 slices of melba toast

5–6 saltine crackers

24 oyster crackers

5 whole-wheat low-fat crackers

15–20 fat-free or baked chips

2 large rice cakes or 6 mini rice cakes

11 soy chips

MOTIVATION FROM TEAM MALLETT

The food plan is a lifestyle diet and I do not feel deprived.

—Lynn Serwin, 40, South Pasadena, California

ENERGY BARS

Beware of these babies because some are really just candy bars in disguise. Often they're marketed as a pick-me-up, especially for that midafternoon slump or on a morning when you don't have time for breakfast. That's true if you choose the right bar. One that's loaded with sugar will only send your sugar levels soaring and then crashing, leaving you feeling worse than before you ate it. Choosing the right bar was a big topic for Team Mallett. Many of them love these bars and are not ready to give them up.

Make sure the bars you choose have no added sugar (which can be disguised as corn syrup and high-fructose corn syrup). It's best if the sugar comes from a natural whole-foods source, such as fruits and nuts. Most bars are high in calories; try sticking with ones around 200 calories. If it has more than that and you're still longing for it, just adjust what you eat for the rest of the day. I'm totally crazy about Lara bar, which is natural and made from whole foods. I often split the bar into two pieces and eat one half in the morning and the other in the afternoon. I also feel good giving my kids these bars in their lunch boxes. My daughter loves the cashew cookie flavor. I know she's getting a good source of protein and omega-3 fatty acids; she thinks mom's letting her eat candy! Imagine the cool mommy points I got for that!

Energy Bars
½ of an approximately 200-calorie bar
½ Lara bar (www.larabar.com)
½ Kookie Karma (www.kookiekarma.com)
½ Balance bar
½ Luna bar
1 Pria bar

Starchy Veggies
1 small baked or boiled potato
1 cup cooked winter (butternut or acorn) and/or summer squash
½ cup yam or sweet potato
½ cup green peas
½ cup of corn or ½ ear of corn
½ cup plantain
½ cup jicama

Beans and Lentils

Note: The following foods are a great source of protein (for example, 1 cup of beans has 12 grams of protein, a perfect choice for vegetarians), but I placed them in the grain section because of their calorie content.

½ cup lentils
⅓ cup baked beans

½ cup cooked beans:
    Black-eyed peas
    Chick peas
    Garbanzo
    Kidney
    Lima beans
    Pinto
    Split peas

FATS

Servings per day: Three

Oils

Note: The following list has the preferred options. 1 teaspoon of the following oils:
    Canola
    Corn
    Flaxseed
    Macadamia
    Olive
    Sesame

Seeds

1 tablespoon or ¼ cup of the following:
    Flaxseed, ground
    Pumpkin
    Sesame
    Sunflower

⅛ an avocado

Nuts

¼ cup or 1 ounce of the following:
    6 almonds
    6 cashews
    10 peanuts
    4 pecan halves
    4 walnut halves

8 olives

Use Sparingly

2 tablespoons reduced-fat salad dressing
1 tablespoon reduced-fat margarine
1 teaspoon regular mayonnaise
2 tablespoons light mayonnaise
1 teaspoon butter
2 tablespoons reduced-fat cream cheese
2 tablespoons reduced-fat sour cream

FREE FOOD

Condiments

Note: As long as you don't eat excessive amounts of the following, there's no need to record them.

Broth, low-sodium

Mustard

Salsa

Soy sauce

Taco sauce

Tomato ketchup

Vinegar

Wine, used in cooking sauce

Worcester sauce

Water

Servings per day: At least eight to ten glasses

Note: Tea and coffee don't count as water!

TREATS

Limit yourself to three or four treats a week. I also recommend that you try and refrain from treats for the first week just to give yourself a little head start. Results keep you going!

Breathe a sigh of relief because, yes, you are allowed treats. Life is too short to completely shut out all the fun foods and drinks. Also, it's not realistic to say that you'll never have a piece of chocolate or a glass of wine again. (I want to meet the gal with that kind of willpower!) Just be aware that if you overeat one day, you should add an extra cardio session that week and watch your portions strictly for the next day. If I overeat, I'm naturally not as hungry the next day and so I eat less. Eventually, your body will get into this rhythm. Even though treats are small, they're dense in calories and often one treat turns into five (or more), especially when you're stressed! Limit yourself to three or four treats a week. Here are some examples:

1 4-ounce glass of wine

1 12-ounce glass of light beer

1½ ounces spirits, either on the rocks or tamed with a diet soda

1 Kashi TLC cookie (oatmeal raisin)

4 Hershey kisses

2 Hershey miniatures

2 ounces angel food cake

1 Vitalicious VitaMuffin, www.vitalicious.com (deep chocolate is my favorite!)

1 bag Kellogg's All-Bran Snack Bites

1 bag Frito-Lay 100-Calorie Mini Bite Sun Chips

½ packet (small bag) of M&M's

11 Stacy's Whole Wheat Bagel chips

I don't recommend that you eat the following foods on a regular basis. But if you happen to find yourself in the hands of temptation, here's a little guide to help you:

Angel food cake: 2 ounces = two grains

Brownie: 1 ounce = one grain and one fat

Cookies, 2 small: 1 ounce = one grain and one to two fats

French fries: 5 ounces = four grains and four fats

Hot dog with bun: 1 = one grain, one protein, and one fat

Ice cream, fat-free or no sugar added: ½ cup = one grain

Ice cream: ½ cup = one grain and two fats

ALCOHOL

Hard liquor has fewer calories than wine or beer, so it may be a better choice if you're going to drink more than one alcoholic beverage. On the other hand, plenty of studies show that red wine is good for your heart.

MOTIVATION FROM TEAM MALLETT

Small meals throughout the day really do help satisfy any cravings to snack on the wrong types of food. I found it helpful to not skip any meal or snack. My body adjusted and I didn't have hunger pains.
—Michele Eaton, 37, Seattle, Washington

Either way, I must stress that you still need to take those extra calories into consideration with your meal plan. If you drink in large quantities on a regular basis, you'll definitely be wearing your booze on your butt!

	Serving (ounces)	Alcohol (grams)	Carbs (grams)	Total Calories
Beer				
Regular	12	13	13	150
Light	12	12	5	100
Non-alcoholic	12	1.5	12	60
Distilled spirits				
80 proof	1.5	14	trace	100
Whisky	1.5	15	trace	105
Wine				
Dry Wine	5	14	2	105
Red or Rose	5	14	2.5	105
Cocktails				
Bloody Mary	5	14	5	115
Daiquiri	4	28	8	220
Tom Collins	7.5	16	3	120
Martini	4	18.5	trace	250

SUMPTUOUS SNACKS

Believe it or not, snacking can help you lose weight and maintain weight loss. That's because by eating a little something between meals you won't be ravenous come lunch or dinner and overeat. It's important to eat every two to three hours to keep your blood sugar levels stable; when your levels dip you get tired, cranky, and devour anything in sight. Plus, skipping meals or snacks puts your body into starvation mode, in which it holds onto fat, making it harder to lose those extra pounds. The trick, however, is to choose the right snacks (chips and dip don't count!). But you'll be surprised at the delicious options you can indulge in. So do yourself a favor and stock up on plenty of snacks. Place them in your bag, your car, your gym locker, your desk, anywhere you can possibly imagine so you're prepared.

Dairy and Protein Based

1 low-fat string cheese

1 Laughing Cow light cheese with three whole-grain crackers

1 Stonyfield Farm Light Smoothie

1 cup low-fat or light yogurt

1 hard-boiled egg dipped in 1 tablespoon light ranch dressing

1 large stalk celery stuffed with 1 tablespoon peanut butter

½ cup fat-free ice cream or frozen yogurt

1 fat-free chocolate pudding cup

1 slice whole-wheat bread with 1 ounce turkey breast and mustard

1 hard-boiled egg with ½ slice toasted wheat bread

1 ounce reduced-fat cheese rolled in 1 ounce deli turkey or chicken meat

1 cup mixed berries with 2 tablespoons plain nonfat yogurt

1 4-inch whole-wheat pita with 1 tablespoon hummus

Veggies and Fruit Snacks

Any piece of fruit

¼ cup low-fat cottage cheese with 1 cup sliced strawberries

1 apple with 1 tablespoon peanut or almond butter

Raw vegetables (especially broccoli, celery, carrots, cauliflower, and red peppers) dipped in hummus

½ cup steamed soybeans (edamame)

1 large stalk celery stuffed with 1 tablespoon peanut butter

1 cup mixed berries with 2 tablespoons plain nonfat yogurt

Energy Bars

½ a 200-calorie energy bar

1 Pria bar = 100 calories

Packaged Snacks

1 100-calorie packet of Wheat Thins

½ ounce baked tortilla chips with 2 tablespoons salsa

20 animal crackers

3 to 4 cups of microwave air-popped popcorn (make sure it has no more than 120 calories and 3 grams of fat)

7 Whole Wheat Triscuits

Cuppa Soups
1 cup low-sodium (less than 350 milligrams) chicken noodle soup with
2 saltine crackers

Nuts
10 almonds
10 cashews

Success Story

Robin Shaddy, 40, mother of two, Papillon, Nebraska

Lost

10 pounds

Two dress sizes

1½ inches off her chest

3 inches off her arms

2 inches off her waist

1½ inches off her hips

2 inches off her legs

10 inches total

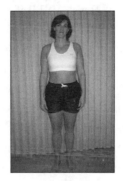

Before

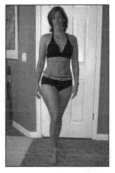

After

ROBIN'S STICK-WITH-IT TIP

*Stick with the food plan. Focus and really concentrate on your portion sizes.
You will not go hungry! The positive change you will feel in a few weeks is unbelievable.
Tracey allows unlimited veggies, so I would add the veggies to my plate first, then fruit,
and then meat. By that time, there was no room on the plate for anything else,
not to mention I was really full after that. This really cut down on my pasta and
bread consumption.*

Gained

Power over her chocolate cravings. *I keep around a bag of Hershey's dark chocolate kisses and eat one after lunch and one after dinner just so I can have my chocolate fix. I was surprised, but it really works.*

• • • • •

Robin Shaddy, 40, realized that losing weight gets harder the older you get. "I had my first child at age 29 and the pregnancy weight came right off," says this married stay-at-home mom. "But when I had my second child at 38, I was still struggling to get the weight off two years later." Those lingering pounds made her feel "miserable, fat, and disgusting" and she was tired all the time. "I had no energy to exercise." Although she'd never been on a formal weight loss plan, Robin tried to slim down by doing her own thing. "I'd exercise here and there, count calories, starve myself, but nothing was getting my metabolism back in the swing of things," she says. Amazingly, Robin had a personal trainer who came to her house once a week, but even that couldn't get her to stick with a fitness program. "I just wasn't motivated and didn't have the energy to do the cardio workouts that I so desperately needed." It was time to change her diet and exercise habits, but she didn't know enough about it. "I really needed a life change and I wanted to learn more about fitness and eating healthy," she says. "I also wanted the motivation to exercise consistently for the rest of my life."

That motivation came in the form of Team Mallett. And it worked. She saw the pounds start to come off and the muscles beneath the fat started to emerge—especially around her middle. "Exercising felt great and I saw my body changing, which felt so awesome and inspired me to keep going," she says. "The more I did it, the easier it got and it was so amazing to see muscle tone."

At first, she thought that the hardest thing about the program was changing her diet. Before, she'd eat donuts, bagels, fast food, and over-sized bowls of cereal. Snacks included cookies, chocolate cake, cup-cakes, and brownies. But seeing her body change motivated her to stick with the food plan, and it actually became her favorite part. "I'm not a very good cook, but the creativity took over so I had variety every week. I started eating foods that I never would have eaten before, and now I love fruits and veggies and drink water instead of soda." She even learned how to deal with her chocolate cravings by eating one dark chocolate Hershey's kiss instead of a pan of brownies or chocolate cake. Robin's whole body felt like it ran more efficiently. "I was amazed by the energy difference when I ate right! I also sleep so much better." Soon enough, friends and family were telling Robin she was shrinking and she agreed. "I felt like I was watching myself get thinner and thinner right before my eyes," she says. "And I was able to get into clothes I hadn't been able to wear for years."

Tracey's influence on Robin's life is huge. Today, she's taking adult ballet classes and has taken up snowboarding. "I'm much more confident and happy. It's an amazing feeling."

TRACEY'S TAKE

One of Robin's biggest goals was to look good in a bikini for a bachelorette party and wedding in Las Vegas. She said that she was nervous and self-conscious wearing a bikini in front of all these women without children. I don't know what she was worrying about—look how amazing she looks. It proves that if you keep your goals alive, you can do it. Even though she's a mom of two, she can still look hot in a bikini. Don't hide behind being a mom; that's just an excuse. Look at Robin, she's your true inspiration!

MOTIVATION FROM TEAM MALLETT

I just realized the other night what a huge impact you have had on my eating. For the first time in my life I have made chili without chocolate cake or brownies accompanying it. I didn't even realize that I had forgot. It also dawned on me that Tracey has had a huge affect on my life. Wow, chili without chocolate cake. Who knew? Thank you for opening my eyes.
—Robin Shaddy, 40, Papillion, Nebraska

CHAPTER 11

NUTRITION 101

THERE'S MORE TO TRIMMING DOWN AND TONING UP THAN breaking a sweat. The other half of the equation is food. Recently, researchers analyzed forty-three weight loss studies from as far back as 1985 and found that just exercising without changing your diet won't help you shed pounds. Your best bet is a combination of working out and healthy eating. No surprise there. But, as you probably know by now, you can't live on rice cakes, grilled chicken, and salad with bland, fat-free dressing on the side. Food with no flavor has, well, no flavor! After weeks of eating what tastes like Styrofoam, you're starving, and that's when you start nibbling here and there and eventually binge.

My solution for this has been to find healthy, low-fat options that taste good and are highly nutritious. When you experiment with food, you'll realize that you can slim down most recipes and find scrumptious, satisfying ways to move toward your goal of a tighter body and a smaller dress size. (I provide recipes in chapter 13.) And when you pay attention to what you're eating and make sure you get the right balance of protein, fat, carbs, and nutrients, you'll actually feel full eating a lot less food. Sounds contradictory, but it's true.

Here's just one example. If I eat a bagel for breakfast, just an hour later my stomach is talking so loud the neighbors can hear it. I'm starving. But if I have whole-wheat toast with some peanut butter (which can equal fewer calories than that plain bagel), the combination of fiber, protein, and fat will keep me full until my morning snack. There's a lot to know about nutrition, but once you do, you can make better choices. Here's a little more about the basics of what's important to include in your diet and why.

PROTEIN

Why do you need protein? Protein, which is found in fish, poultry, meat, dairy, and some grains, is essential for muscle repair and the complete maintenance of your body. It makes hormones and helps your immune system. It can also help you shed pounds. Here's why. Protein requires more energy to digest than carbs and fat, so you actually burn more calories eating it. Protein also helps preserve and build lean muscle tissue while you trim down. And muscle burns more calories than fat—even while you're just sitting on your bum watching television.

If your body doesn't get enough protein and important essential amino acids daily, it takes what it needs from existing muscles. That means you're actually losing valuable fat-burning tissue! Protein-rich foods also help to slow down the absorption of glucose into the bloodstream. This keeps your blood sugar levels consistent, which helps suppress hunger. Now do you see why it's so important to eat protein at each meal? Luckily, you can choose from lots of different foods—just watch out for meats with excess fats.

In this section I describe the different sources of protein.

WHO KNEW?

Besides water, protein is the most plentiful substance in the body. It makes up your muscles, eyes, individual cells, and skin!

Meat and Fish

Chicken, turkey, salmon, and white fish are perfect, low-fat choices. But steer clear of duck, which has a high fat content, and choose only very lean cuts of beef and pork. Most grocers have select prime cuts, and though they're usually more expensive, your heart and body are worth it. Salmon is a great protein option because it contains omega-3 fatty acids (which I discuss in a few pages) and various B vitamins, vitamin D, potassium, and selenium. It's also low in mercury—a key fact when shopping for fish. Others in that category are haddock, cod, tilapia, sole, most shellfish, and canned albacore tuna. Swordfish, king mackerel, and shark have a high mercury content and should be eaten in moderation.

Eggs

The media has given eggs—specifically their yolks—a raw deal by blaming them for high cholesterol. Yes, they do contain it, but if you have normal cholesterol levels and limit your intake of other fats, you can safely eat an egg a day. For those with high cholesterol, eat no more than four eggs a week. Egg whites are a great source of protein with no saturated fat, and I think there's nothing better than a veggie-packed egg white omelet. I would definitely recommend this as your order of choice at a restaurant for breakfast. Something else I love is making a batch of hard-boiled eggs on Sunday and having them in the refrigerator all week to grab and eat. (Can't think of a better and more filling 70-calorie snack.)

Plus, eggs have lots of other crucial nutrients such as folate, vitamins E and B12, omega-3 and omega-6 fatty acids, and antioxidants such as lutein. The latter is important for good eye health and preventing age-related macular degeneration, one of the top causes of vision loss among older Americans.

Whey

I love whey protein because it's quickly absorbed by the body and gives you antioxidant protection. You can easily add it to your diet by mixing whey protein powder into smoothies, cereal, juice, or water. It is instant high-quality protein that you don't have to cook—that's my kind of food. Plus, whey protein tastes good.

Just be careful when choosing your whey powder. Read the label to make sure that it has virtually no fat, contains whey protein isolates (which are absorbed faster than other forms), and is microfiltered, a method that keeps the proteins intact. Because whey is digested quickly, it allows the amino acids to repair the muscles that are building lean muscle mass. Try a whey protein smoothie after you exercise in the morning, and you may notice less post-workout soreness. In my opinion, whey protein is an integral part of your weight loss system.

Soy

Soy (a.k.a. soy beans) is a great protein option, especially for vegetarians, and has become popular in the last few years. At any grocery store, you'll find tofu, edamame, soy burgers, soy butter, and soy sausages, so there's no longer any excuse to scrimp on protein if you don't eat meat. Soybeans also contain isoflavones, a type of phytoestrogen, that are considered by some nutritionists and physicians to be useful in the prevention

MOTIVATION FROM TEAM MALLETT

After six weeks of eating healthily, I indulged in nachos and tequitos at a family event and got sick to my stomach! My body was rejecting bad greasy food. It wasn't worth it anyway, because I love my new healthy food plan!
—Alison Fukomoto, 29, Santa Monica, California

of cancer. Some studies have even found that soy protein can help lower bad (LDL) cholesterol a modest amount. One controversial aspect to soy is that some researchers believe it may put breast cancer patients at a greater risk for a recurrence of the disease, because the phytoestrogens found in soy can stimulate cell growth. (Breast cancer patients should discuss this with their doctor.)

DAIRY

Dairy foods are important for women because they contain lots of protein and calcium, which we need to ward off the bone-thinning disease osteoporosis. According to the National Osteoporosis Foundation, an estimated ten million Americans—eight million women and two million men—have osteoporosis and another thirty-four million have low bone mass, which increases their risk for this disease. People typically lose bone as they age, so you have to do everything you can to keep yours strong. (Exercise helps big time.) The daily recommended amount of calcium for women under 50 is 1,000 mg a day and for those over 50 is 1,200 mg. You can reach this through calcium-rich foods such as milk, cottage cheese, and fruit.

Here are some examples of the calcium content in everyday foods:

Part-skim ricotta cheese: 1 cup provides 669 mg
Yogurt: 8 ounces provides 415 mg
Milk, 2%: 1 cup provides 285 mg
Swiss cheese: 1 ounce provides 224 mg
Cottage cheese: 1 cup provides 126 mg

Calcium may also help ward off other diseases. One new study found that calcium and vitamin D may reduce your risk of colon cancer. And some research shows that dairy foods may help you lose weight. Plus, they can help you feel like you're indulging even when you're not; food such as low-fat yogurt has a creamy feel and sweet taste. Add a drop of chocolate to your milk and you'll satisfy a chocolate craving and a calcium requirement.

VEGGIES

On my food plan (chapter 10), you'll see that you can eat an unlimited amount of veggies. Yes, you read that correctly: unlimited! Sure, it's rare to find a food you can eat until your heart's content, but it's also rare to find people who overeat veggies. Let's get real here: If you're overweight, you didn't get that way by eating too many carrots. In fact, most of us eat a lot fewer vegetables each day than what the USDA suggests for a healthy diet. So go on, fill up your plate! Just don't douse those veggies in heavy, rich sauces.

One reason veggies are so good? They contain vitamins A, C, and E and several key minerals. Plus, veggies have fiber and lots of water so they fill you up on very few calories. They're also a great source of anti-oxidants, compounds in food that help prevent the oxidation that naturally happens to cells in our body. The American Dietetic Association describes it like this: "Just like rust on a car, oxidation can cause damage to cells and may contribute to aging." This cell damage is believed to lead to an array of diseases from cancer to Alzheimer's, so loading up on antioxidants is a great idea. Antioxidants are also believed to help boost your immune system and keep your skin looking young and radiant. Brightly colored and dark green veggies typically contain the most powerful antioxidants.

FRUITS

If you have a sweet tooth, you'll be surprised at how satisfying fruit can be. I'm not saying it'll replace a good piece of chocolate cake (I wish!), but it can take the edge off when you're longing for something tasty. The best thing to do is to eat what's in season in your area because it usually is the freshest and least expensive and tastes best. Think peaches and plums in summer, pears and apples in fall, and oranges and grapefruit in winter. But unlike veggies, fruits aren't something you can eat in unlimited quantities. I've had several clients who couldn't understand why they weren't losing weight, but when we discussed their diet, we realized that they thought they could eat all the fruit they wanted. Nope. It still has calories and its own natural sugar. So enjoy but don't go hog wild.

(The American Dietetic Association recommends eating about two cups daily.) One of my favorite treats is to cut up an apple, add a dash of cinnamon and a tiny teaspoon of brown sugar, and microwave it for one to two minutes. I swear, it's like apple pie without the fat. For simple-to-make smoothies, stash bananas and grapes in the freezer and buy frozen berries.

When you're talking about dried fruit, make sure to keep your portions super small, such as two tablespoons of raisins. Dried fruit is a more concentrated version of fresh fruit, so it's higher in calories. That said, it's a great substitute for candy and a sweet way to top yogurt, oatmeal, cold cereal, and salads.

> **WHO KNEW?**
>
> A whopping 73 percent of Americans say they eat junk food because it's convenient. Make healthy food convenient by cutting up fruits and veggies and having them at eye level in your refrigerator.

CARBOHYDRATES (GRAINS)

In recent years, carbohydrates have received a bad rap. The media and lots of fad diets have led people to believe that carbs will plump you up, so banning pasta, rice, and bread will slim you down. That's rubbish. Our brains and muscles need a certain amount of carbs to supply us with the energy to work out and lead our busy lives. And the liver needs carbs to keep its glycogen reserves well stocked. That's one reason why our body craves carbs—especially when we deprive it of them.

But not all carbs are created equal. The various kinds are broken down by our bodies differently and can affect how much food we eat by the rate at which the sugar enters our bloodstream. Here's how it works. There are three simple sugars: glucose (found in starches), fructose (from fruits and honey), and galactose (found in dairy products). Fructose and galactose must first be converted to glucose in your liver before slowly trickling into your bloodstream. This happens at a very slow rate (often referred to as low glycemic index). Because most carbs in the dairy and fruit category contain these kinds of sugars, they generally keep your energy levels balanced, which essentially will keep you feeling fuller longer between meals.

On the flip side, glucose-rich foods such as bread and pasta bypass the liver and practically sprint into the bloodstream. That's why after eating a slice of white bread, you get a sudden surge of energy. Unfortunately, what quickly goes up must quickly go down, leaving you even more hungry than you were before you ate. One way to slow down this process is to pair the carbs with some protein, such as chicken with your pasta or turkey on wheat bread. My point here? Welcome carbs back to the dinner table, but just make sure they're the right carbs.

FIBER

Carbs are also important because most of them contain fiber, and let's just say fiber can be your best friend when it comes to weight loss. I personally think it's the best-kept secret for slimming down. Fiber keeps you full longer, and we all know that it's much easier to avoid the cookie jar or drive-through when you're full. Fiber works its magic because it moves through the body more slowly than other foods such as highly processed ones (for example, cookies and white bread), so you're satisfied longer. In fact, a study that appeared a few years ago in the *Journal of the American Heart Association* found that people who ate a high-fiber diet weighed an average of 8 pounds less compared to those who ate a low-fiber diet.

Dietary fiber is a general term for indigestible parts of plant foods. The two basic kinds of fiber are soluble and insoluble. You can find soluble fiber in oat bran, flaxseed, apples, oranges, and nuts. It dissolves in water to form a soft gel in your intestines; this means it can pick up stuff in there that could harm your health, such as cholesterol and fatty acids, while helping regulate insulin levels. (In English, it will keep you feeling satisfied for longer periods of time so you don't overindulge in extra food.)

Tracey's Tip

Add a tablespoon of freshly ground flaxseed or a handful of nuts to your cereal or smoothies.

Insoluble fiber is cellulose, the main fiber in the cell walls of all plants. This kind absorbs water, but it doesn't dissolve in it, so you need to drink more water when eating large amounts of fiber. Eating insoluble fiber helps alleviate colon and bowel problems, and when your colon and bowels are clean, you may experience less bloating and less puffiness in the lower part of your abs. The thin outer husks of whole grains such as rice, wheat, and oats (called bran) are insoluble fiber and rich sources of B vitamins and minerals. Fiber-rich foods can also lower blood fat levels and keep your digestive system running more smoothly.

Some fiber-rich foods to stock up on are apples, bananas, citrus fruits, pears, and strawberries; asparagus, broccoli, brussels sprouts, carrots, cauliflower, corn, green beans, and sweet potatoes; cooked beans, lentils, oat bran, oatmeal, rice bran, nuts, and seeds. A healthy recommended daily intake of fiber a day is 25–35 grams. However, if you haven't been eating fiber, don't rush to eat this much overnight. Instead, slowly add fiber to your diet to avoid constipation and bloating. And remember that the more fiber you eat, the more water you need to consume, too.

WHO KNEW?

Steel-cut oatmeal, not instant, is one of the healthiest carbs around. It's low on the glycemic load scale and has a high fiber content, so it enters your bloodstream slowly and keeps you full for hours. Eat it for breakfast and those midmorning hunger pangs will be a thing of the past.

FATS

Like carbs, fats used to have a bad reputation in the world of weight loss. Remember that craze a few years back when everything was labeled low fat or no fat? We all just got a lot fatter because these foods still had the same number of calories and often had more sugar than the original products. I was guilty of this back in the early 90s. I was a dancer doing musical theater and needed to keep my pathetically low show weight consistent. I honestly thought if I ate everything nonfat I wouldn't get fat. I'd fill up on things such as huge bags of pretzels and rice cakes in one go. Well, like many people, I was wrong—I messed up my digestive system and couldn't understand why my weight was going up, not down. Over the years I've realized that weight loss is as simple as calories in and calories out. And if you eat excessively, those excess calories go on your hips and butt whether the calories have fat in them or not!

Fortunately, healthy fat is no longer taboo. And that's a good thing because your body can't function without it. Fat is a high source of fuel. One gram of fat is 9 calories, compared to protein and carbs, which are each 4 calories. It also gives texture and flavor to foods and helps us feel content after we eat. In addition, it protects

WHO KNEW?

Bad fats such as lard and butter are solid at room temperature. Healthy fats such as olive oil and canola oil are liquid. You have no excuse not to tell them apart!

our organs, aids in the development of cell membranes and hormones, and insulates our body's organs. However, it's important that you understand the right kinds of fat your body needs for health and disease prevention.

Good Fats

Let's start with the good fats. Unsaturated fats are mostly found in plant sources such as nuts, seeds, vegetable oils, and avocados. They decrease low-density lipoprotein (LDL), also known as the bad cholesterol. (I describe them as artery cleaners to my clients.) They also increase high-density lipoprotein (HDL), the good cholesterol.

Good-for-you fats slow down the digestion of carbohydrates and their release into your system. As a result, they keep insulin levels lower, so you don't get a sugar rush and crash that leaves you starving. The good fats release the cholecystokinin (CCK) hormone from your stomach, which sends a message to your brain that you're satisfied and don't need to eat more. Without that message, you would continue to chow down even when your stomach is full, and that's a surefire recipe for packing on the pounds. Fats also help your body absorb vitamins such as A, D, E, and K and calcium, and they nourish your skin, hair, nerves, and mucous membranes. That's why going on a no-fat, low-calorie, I'm-just-eating-carrots diet makes your hair look parched and brittle and your skin look dry and sallow. (Women with eating disorders such as anorexia often have hair and skin that looks this way.) The American Heart Association's Nutrition Committee strongly advises these fat guidelines for healthy Americans over age 2:

- Limit total fat intake to less than 25–35 percent of your total calories each day.
- Limit saturated fat intake to less than 7 percent of total daily calories.
- Limit trans fat intake to less than 1 percent of total daily calories.
- The remaining fat should come from sources of monounsaturated and polyunsaturated fats such as nuts, seeds, fish, and vegetable oils.
- Limit cholesterol intake to less than 300 milligrams per day, for most people. If you have coronary heart disease or your LDL

cholesterol level is 100 mg/dL or greater, limit your cholesterol intake to less than 200 milligrams a day.

Omega-3 fats are also known as essential fatty acids (EFAs). They're called essential because our body cannot produce these fats and the only way to get them is through our diet. They're found mainly in oily fish such as salmon, sardine, mackerel, herring, and trout. Flaxseeds are also a great choice, especially if you're a vegetarian.

Another good fat is omega-6 fat, which you'll find in dark green vegetables; nuts and seeds such as sunflower, pumpkin, sesame, and flax; and olive and canola oil. EFAs are important for brain function, for memory, and for maintaining healthy hair, skin, and nails. They're also believed to reduce blood pressure and the risk of blot clots. Other studies say they may help relieve depression—one reason why I think of them as oiling the brain. Not only do they affect your mood but they help with memory function. Could there be a better food for a busy, multitasking woman like you? I didn't think so.

Bad Fats

The bad fats are saturated fats, which are in oxidized, hydrogenated, or heat-processed foods. You'll find them in fried foods, margarine, vegetable shortening, and processed items such as cookies, biscuits, and pie crusts. Even foods that seem healthy, such as cereals and granola bars, can have them. Try and stay away from these saturated fats, which are found in full-fat milk, fatty meats, and tropical oils (coconut oil).

The worst kind of saturated fat is trans fat. It's so bad that in the last two years, the FDA has required that all trans fat content be specified on food labels. Some restaurants—even fast food joints—are phasing out their use of trans fats. Trans fats are formed when vegetable oil is converted from a liquid fat to a solid. This lengthens its shelf life so that

MOTIVATION FROM TEAM MALLETT

I feel much better now that I'm drinking water instead of soda,
and eating less is easier on my digestive system.
My body feels like it's running more efficiently.
— Robin Shaddy, 40, Papillion, Nebraska

processed foods can last longer, but it also boosts your risk for heart disease. I've heard experts say that reducing trans fat consumption could prevent up to 1,200 cases of coronary heart disease and save between 250 and 500 lives over the next three years.

The American Heart Association emphasizes that you should eat vegetables, fruits, whole grain/high fiber foods, fat-free and low-fat dairy products, lean meats, and fish, and that you should limit the amount of trans fat, saturated fat, and cholesterol you consume. This is easy to do if you stop munching on food that comes out of a box or a bag. You'll know if something contains trans fats if you see partially hydrogenated and shortening on the ingredient list. Also skip the butter and margarine and cook with olive oil and canola oil.

ALCOHOL

Did you know that alcohol is metabolized as sugar and if you drink it excessively the body stores it as fat? Yup! Now you know why men and women who drink a lot of alcohol have beer bellies. Drinking too much of the sudsy stuff is the closest they're going to get to a six pack!

Just one 4-ounce serving of alcohol is considered two food exchanges of fat. The typical serving of wine at a bar or restaurant is 6 ounces, and who stops at just one glass? I'm not saying don't drink. But you have to watch your alcohol consumption just like you watch food portions.

DID YOU KNOW?

Red wine gets its rich, ruby hue from antioxidants called polyphenols, and these compounds may be good for your heart. A study in the *European Journal of Clinical Nutrition* found that a single glass of alcohol-free red wine relaxes the arteries of people with atherosclerosis. This may help lower blood pressure and ultimately reduce your risk of heart attack and stroke.

WATER

Water is more than a drink we tote around in little bottles. Drinking enough is essential for life and for making sure your body functions at its best. Water is to your body what motor oil is to your car—it helps it run efficiently. Water regulates your metabolism, helps with digestion, and flushes rubbish out of the body. It helps all your vital organs function. It transports valuable nutrients to and from working muscles and is directly responsible for maintaining body temperature. In fact, 70 percent of your body is water.

But that's not the only reason why water is super important for weight loss. A common myth is that drinking too much water causes water retention, but the opposite is true. When your body is dehydrated, it holds onto water, which can cause bloating and puffiness. When you're dehydrated— either from sweating too much or not drinking enough—you often mistake thirst for hunger. To make yourself feel better, you reach for food when water would do the trick.

WHO KNEW?

- 75 percent of Americans are chronically dehydrated.
- In 37 percent of Americans, the thirst mechanism is so weak that it is mistaken for hunger.
- Even mild dehydration slows your metabolism down by as much as 3 percent.
- One glass of water quelled the midnight hunger pains for almost 100 percent of dieters in a University of Washington study.
- Lack of water is the number-one trigger of daytime fatigue.
- Preliminary research indicates that eight to ten glasses of water a day could significantly ease back and joint pain for up to 80 percent of sufferers.
- A mere 2 percent drop in body water can trigger fuzzy short-term memory, trouble with basic math, and difficulty focusing on the computer screen or on a printed page.
- Drinking five glasses of water daily decreases the risk of colon cancer by 45 percent, the risk of breast cancer by 79 percent, and the risk of bladder cancer by 50 percent. (Are you drinking the amount of water you should drink every day?)
- Your muscles are 70 percent water.

I recommend that you plan water into your daily schedule so that you're drinking it consistently. Don't wait until you're thirsty because that's a sign of dehydration. (Other signs include difficulty concentrating, dizziness, headaches, muscle spasms, constipation, water retention, fatigue, irritability, and dark urine.)

We all love coffee and tea, but you can't count this as water consumption. They're diuretics, so if you're one of those people who drinks coffee through an intravenous drip, I suggest you try cutting down to two or three cups a day and swap that cream for skimmed milk or, gulp, try going black. I'm a confessed tea-aholic (I *am* British) and have no intention of giving up my lovely cuppa. However, I do limit myself or opt for the herbal, caffeine-free variety.

If you find drinking huge amounts of water difficult, try some flavored water. Just check that it has no added sugar or artificial sweeteners and no calories. A favorite of mine is called Hint. It's pure water with, as the name implies, just a hint of natural flavor from fruit. You can also fill a big pitcher with water and drop in some lemon, orange, or grapefruit juice. Even cucumbers or strawberries taste delicious and give water a refreshing, spa-like taste.

Besides keeping you slim, drinking more water can also help you improve your skin. I used to be a diet soda girl, downing an embarrassing number of cans per day. But once I gave that up and tried drinking enough water, my acne-prone skin cleared up. It makes you wonder how many more illnesses and disease could be prevented from just drinking water that the body craves and needs.

GOING ORGANIC

Organic foods are grown with fewer chemicals and pesticides, so they're better for you and the earth. Having kids really made me take a second look at what I was putting in my mouth and theirs. I saw their bodies as clean slates and realized I didn't want to fill them with chemicals. I choose to buy only organic products whenever possible, and luckily these foods are available beyond the health food store. In fact, the organic food market has grown 15–20 percent annually for the last ten years. Just make sure to look at labels carefully. If a product sports the green and white USDA Organic seal, that means it contains at least 95 percent organic ingredients. Those with 70–95 percent can be labeled "made with organic ingredients" but can't carry the seal, and those with less than 70 percent can only mention their organic components in the ingredient list.

SUGAR AND SWEETENERS

Ah, sugar. It's so, well, sweet. Natural sugar from foods such as fruit are not what you have to worry about. It's the hidden sugars that you need to run from. Not only are they bad for your health, but they'll burn through your daily calorie budget fast. Some of the big sugar companies boast about the fact that sugar has only 15 calories per teaspoon. But have you actually looked at a teaspoon lately? It's not that big. And the more sugar you consume, the more it takes to get the sweet taste you're craving.

To figure out how many teaspoons you're eating, look at the food labels and divide the sugar amount in grams by 4. For example, if a serving has 12 grams of sugar, you will be consuming 3 teaspoons of sugar.

One of the worst sweeteners is high-fructose corn syrup (HFCS). You should avoid it completely if you're trying to slim down and stay that way. "It was introduced into our food supply about forty years ago," says Phil Wood, Ph.D., director of the division of genomics at the University of Alabama and author of *How Fat Works*. "Today it represents more than 40 percent of the caloric sweeteners added to foods and beverages and it's used in everything from bread to soda to ketchup." The problem? HFCS enters the bloodstream more quickly than other types of sugar. The hormonal and chemical changes that occur make you feel even hungrier, so you eat more without feeling satisfied. In fact, research shows that the increased use of HFCS in this country mirrors the rapid increase in obesity and may play a role. Start reading food labels carefully and keep foods with HFCS out of your shopping cart and cupboard.

WHO KNEW?

Despite efforts to turn the problem of obesity around, the Centers for Disease Control and Prevention (CDC) says it's getting worse. Our obesity rates have nearly doubled from an estimated 15 percent in 1980 to nearly 30 percent today.

One of the most frequent questions I get asked is, what sweetener do I recommend? Real sugar in moderation. I'm not a fan of the artificial stuff. Lots of products with aspartame carry a cancer warning from a preliminary study with rats linked to an increase in malignant tumors and other cancers. That's another big reason why I gave up my addiction to diet soda. Canada has even banned aspartame in foods. I also think fake sweeteners perpetuate your craving for sweet things and it's better to get over your sweet tooth.

I suggest going cold turkey for two weeks and try to avoid as much sugar as possible. You will be amazed how sickly sweet it tastes after a few weeks without it. It worked for me. Now that I have kids, I'm in that world of attending frequent birthday parties and special days at school. It seems like every week there's another occasion filled with candy and cake, but having worked through my sweet tooth, I can accompany my kids to those fun events without ruining my healthy eating plan.

FOOD PORTIONS

Can you believe that portion sizes have doubled in the past twenty years? Two cups of pasta used to be the norm. Now it is common to see at least four cups on your plate at an Italian restaurant. Sodas during the 1950s and 1960s were about 7 ounces, compared with 12 to 64 ounces these days. At the movies, popcorn was once about 5 to 6 cups; now a large bucket with butter flavor contains up to 20 cups and 1,640 calories.

Check out how we've grown. Twenty years ago:

WHO KNEW?

The average American woman went from weighing 140 pounds in 1960 to 164 pounds in 2002. Today, more than half the women between the ages of 20 and 39 are overweight or obese.

- A muffin was 1.5 ounces and had 210 calories. Today's 5-ounce muffin has 500 calories.
- An average-sized cookie was 55 calories. Today, a large cookie has about 275 calories.
- A bagel was 3 inches in diameter and had 140 calories. Today's 6-inch bagel has 350 calories.
- A 2.4 ounce portion of French fries had 210 calories. Today's 6.9-ounce portion of French fries has 610 calories.
- A cheeseburger had 333 calories. Today's fast food cheeseburger has 590 calories.

Tracey's Tip

In Japan, dinner plates are the size of our bread plates, which may explain why Japan doesn't have an obesity problem. Copy this culture and use smaller plates and cups at meals. This will naturally stop you from piling on huge portions.

The key to eating healthy and understanding what your body truly needs is to be able to eyeball correct portions. Calorie counting is just too time consuming and unrealistic for most of us. Who has the time to keep referring to a book of foods and then hoping you can find the specific brand? I never made a good walking calculator; I'm more of a visual person. The visuals I've created are an easy reference, but I recommend that you also use measuring cups, spoons, and a scale. These will be your new best friends.

The Portion Plate

I love The Portion Plate (www.theportionplate.com) because it gives you a quick reference of what your plate should look like at mealtimes:

- One-half should be fruits and vegetables
- One-fourth should be whole grains
- One-fourth should be lean protein

The graphics on the plate show you portion equivalents, as follows:

- Tennis ball = 1 fruit serving
- Cassette tape = 1 slice bread, presliced (1 serving of grain)
- Computer mouse = 4-ounce serving of uncooked meat or fish (4 servings of protein) or a potato (1 serving of grain)
- 1 yogurt container = 8 ounces (1 serving of dairy)
- 1 baseball = 1 cup raw vegetables (1 serving of veggies)
- ½ baseball = ½ cup of cooked vegetables (1 serving of veggies)
- 4 stacked dimes = 1 fat serving or 1 ounce of cheese (1 dairy)

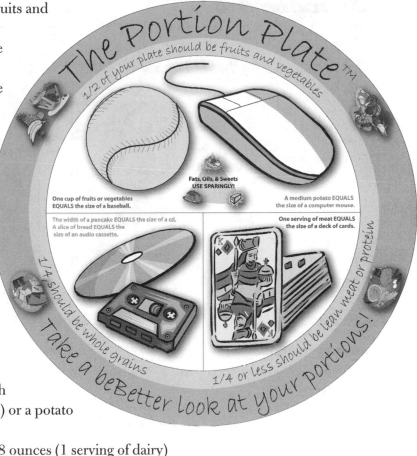

The Portion Plate™

1/2 of your plate should be fruits and vegetables

One cup of fruits or vegetables EQUALS the size of a baseball.

Fats, Oils, & Sweets USE SPARINGLY!

A medium potato EQUALS the size of a computer mouse.

The width of a pancake EQUALS the size of a cd. A slice of bread EQUALS the size of an audio cassette.

One serving of meat EQUALS the size of a deck of cards.

1/4 should be whole grains

1/4 or less should be lean meat or protein

Take a beBetter look at your portions!

QUICK HAND VISUALS

- 2 fists = 1 cup
- 1 fist = 1/2 cup
- Palm of your hand = 3 ounces (a cooked serving of meat, or 3 proteins)
- Thumb = 1 ounce (a piece of cheese)

Success Story

....

Randi Hsu, 42, mother of two, Short Hills, New Jersey

Lost

17 pounds

One dress size

3 inches off her chest

3 inches off arms

6½ inches off her waist

5½ inches off her hips

4 inches off her legs

22 inches total

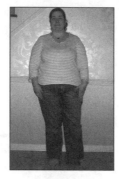 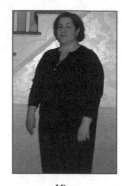

Before   After

Gained

A sense of pride. *This program has allowed me to become a more positive woman. I know I can live a healthy life and be a good role model for my daughter.*

• • • • •

Randi Hsu was about to turn 42 and was determined not to spend another birthday feeling bad about her body. Although she'd carried an extra 10–15 pounds for most of her life, Randi had gained a lot of weight while pregnant with her first child—now 10 years old—and never lost it. "I was depressed and disappointed in myself about being out of shape and overweight," says this mother of two from Short Hills, New Jersey. "I felt so horrible that there were nights that I cried about it."

Although she'd tried many diets and plans in the past, *Sexy in 6* seemed different. "I could tell it would teach me how to make lifestyle changes that I could live with forever, not temporary changes that I'd eventually give up," she says. Soon, Tracey wasn't the only one with energy to burn. "This program taught me that exercise can really be fun and invigorating," says Randi. "I actually get disappointed when there's a day that I don't have time to do more than forty minutes of a cardio workout!"

Randi also revamped her diet. Before the program, she typically ate lots of bagels, muffins, sandwiches, and take-out as well as processed foods such as crackers and cheese curls. "I often finished what was left on my kids' plates and ate standing up," she recalls. She said good-bye to those detrimental behaviors and instead learned new ones. "I'd experiment with different veggies and realized that they could add lots of flavor and really fill me up," she says. "The most amazing thing about this food plan is that you can eat and feel full, and still lose weight!" Another nice surprise was an improved relationship with her husband. "In the past, he'd get frustrated when I'd try every fad diet out there," she says. "This time he saw that I was doing it the right way—no gimmicks—and how much of an effort I was making, and it really helped our relationship."

Most days Randi did well and stuck with the program, and soon her stomach looked flatter and her face wasn't as puffy. But even when she did slip, she kept a positive outlook. "I'd remind myself that I went from not moving at all and eating mindlessly to paying attention to how and what I am eating and moving as much as possible," says Randi. "I tried to stay focused on the healthy food plan and squeezing exercise in when I could."

Although she loved how people told her how different she looked and raved about her clearer complexion, the best compliment came from her 10-year-old daughter. "She actually said that I looked hip, which believe it or not, meant a lot to me since I live in a town where the moms look like they stepped out of *Vogue* when they pick up their kids at school," says Randi. "Plus, my skin looks so much better. It's not dry and my coloring is better."

Her next goal is to lose an additional 70 pounds. "I have a long journey ahead of me, but now I see that I can become healthy and fit," she says. "Tracey has taught me that it's never too late to try to change the

RANDI'S STICK-WITH-IT TIP

Get organized. Write your workouts into your calendar even if you can only exercise thirty minutes that day, and figure out your meals ahead of time.

way you look and feel." This year, Randi celebrated her birthday feeling slimmer and fitter than ever.

TRACEY'S TAKE

Randi's story speaks out to millions of women who are desperately unhappy living in their own body. One of the first e-mails I received from Randi was almost a plea for help; I could feel the sadness in her words. She knew she needed to lose weight but didn't know how. The guilt of wanting to be a good role model for her daughter was weighing heavy on her shoulders. I know it's not been easy for her, but now she has the confidence in herself to keep going. *Sexy in 6* gave her the jump-start she so desperately needed. Words can't express how proud I am of her; she is now on the road to a new life of feeling confident and being able to look in the mirror and say, "I look good." Now that's a success story if I've ever heard one!

MOTIVATION FROM TEAM MALLETT

I'm really enjoying the way the plan makes me feel.
Following it has taken away my interest in cheating.
— *Liz Price, 37, South Pasadena, California*

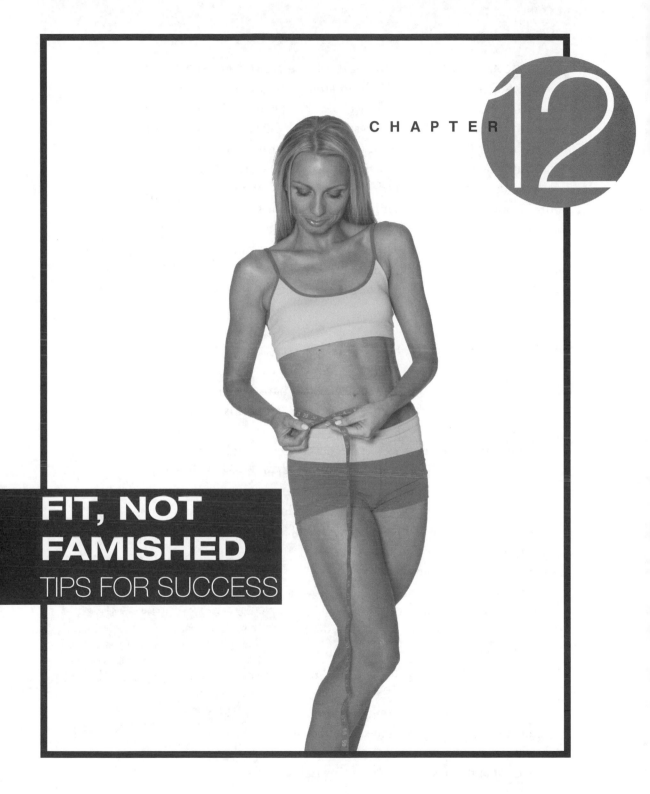

CHAPTER 12

FIT, NOT FAMISHED

TIPS FOR SUCCESS

L OOK, I LOVE FOOD AS MUCH AS THE NEXT GAL, BUT I ALSO know that certain foods head straight to my butt. I've worked hard for my fit body and have to work equally hard to maintain it. But I also like to eat, and I refuse to subsist on rice cakes, steamed carrots, and no-fat everything. I also refuse to sit at home instead of going out to eat—something I think of as a lovely treat. As a result, I've come up with some great tricks and tips that keep me, as this chapter title says, fit not famished. Some may not work for you, but others will. Just like my workouts, you can choose those you like and that fit your lifestyle. If you discover any great tips you'd like to share, feel free to e-mail them to me at tracey@traceymallett.com.

WHO KNEW?

Chocolate is believed to boost endorphin levels in the brain, which may be the explanation for the feel-good factor chocoholics get.

MALLETT'S MEAL POINTERS

- Go low fat. Eat individual food items that have 3 grams or less of total fat per serving. Fish high in omega-3 fatty acids are an exception to this rule.
- Enjoy unlimited veggies. You can never have enough veggies in your diet, especially because they're so rich in disease-fighting vitamins, minerals, and antioxidants. When possible, stick with certified organic veggies—pesticides can interfere with your ability to lose body fat. Eat a minimum of five servings of veggies a day.
- Eat every three hours. Keep your metabolism on fire with a constant flow of energy from healthy foods. Eat protein with each meal, and snack to keep your sugar levels consistent and stop those sugar dips that send you searching for a candy bar.
- Don't skip meals. You won't lose any more weight by skipping meals; in fact, it will only leave you hungrier and force you to overeat at the next meal. How many times have

Tracey's Tip

The worst thing you can do is pick out of the fridge, instead of placing food on a plate. A nibble here and a nibble there add up, though we conveniently forget those bites we took. I know because I'm a picker—a habit I learned from my mother. I grew up watching her hands wander in the kitchen like an octopus and have had to work hard to reform my ways!

you starved yourself before going out for a nice meal and ended up eating like a horse and rolling out of the restaurant feeling guilty? Enough said.

- Reduce caffeinated drinks. Coffee, black tea, colas, and chocolate are in this category. As an English girl, I love tea, so this is a hard one for me, too. Just know that I'm struggling right along with you, baby!

- Limit refined carbs and processed white flours. This means white pastas, white rice, white bread, sugars, and syrups.

- Go whole grain. Whole grain foods such as beans, lentil soups, steel-cut oats, and whole-wheat cereal absorb more water in your stomach, making you feel full faster and satisfied longer. They also prevent sugar spikes, decreasing the chances of midafternoon munchies.

- Say so long to your deep fryer. Deep-fried foods of any kind are a big no-no. Always broil, bake, or grill. If you're preparing a stir-fry or you need to sauté some veggies, use a tiny amount of olive oil.

- Eliminate high-fat desserts. All I can say is "empty calories." They have no nutritional value and loads of calories. Stay away!

- Know the difference between good fat and bad fat. Omega-3 fats found in foods such as fish oils, flaxseeds, and olive oil should be an essential part of your diet. Our bodies need fat to function!

- Get your fill of water. Drink water with every meal. It not only helps with digestion but will give you a feeling of being full. You should consume eight glasses of water every day.

Tracey's Tips

- Buy good nonstick cooking pans and a steamer. They reduce the amount of oil you need to cook with.
- Always eat breakfast. Never go out the door without consuming food!
- From the time you wake up until you go to sleep, eat at least every three hours. Set your clock if you're finding this a hard task until your body naturally tells you.
- Make your home a safe zone. Keep yourself away from temptation by removing tempting foods from your kitchen. Get rid of high-processed packaged foods and always have healthy treats nearby.

EATING OUT

I love eating out, partly because we rarely did it when I was a little girl. In our little town, the only food joints offered good old English fish and chips (a.k.a. fat- and grease-filled heart attack food). On this side of the ocean, eating out is practically a professional sport. We do it much more than people did decades ago and we're plumping up as a result. Remember when you thought dining out was a treat, maybe for a special occasion? Those were the days. Today, with our hectic lives, going to one of the many local restaurants seems easier than stepping into the kitchen.

The first problem is that portion sizes are huge—double what they were just twenty years ago—and you can't see the hidden fats or sugars in the foods. To make matters worse, when you're at a restaurant, your frame of mind is more relaxed and you tend to socialize more. You mindlessly eat, and before you know it the bread basket and your enormous entrée are gone. Temptation is a huge problem in restaurants, especially after a glass of vino (or two or three). Suddenly, you become less concerned about the size of your thighs.

Also, if your pals are chowing down, you often think, why not? Secretly, they want you to eat—I mean indulge—alongside them. Somehow your pigging out soothes their guilt about what they're eating. (As humans we like to do things in packs.) When it gets to that point, I usually try and take a bathroom break or refocus the attention onto someone else. I also take a moment to concentrate on how much better I'm going to feel if I don't overeat. Another trick: I wear my tight hipster jeans as a constant reminder not to overindulge—after all, popping the button or a seam would be embarrassing. Try it and I promise you will think twice!

You have to be savvy and prepared for land mines when you enter a restaurant. Here are some tips:

1. **Do not go to dinner starving.** Temptation will probably get the better of you. Instead, eat a piece of fruit or some veggies about an hour before you go out.

2. **Order your meal—or at least decide what you'll order—before you have an alcoholic drink.** People tend to make better choices and have more willpower before they have alcohol in their system.

3. **Take the bread basket away.** The temptation is far too strong when soft, warm rolls and creamy butter are right in front of your nose. Move it out of your reach or say good-bye to it altogether by asking the waiter to take it away. This could blow all your hard work for the week and it's not worth it!

4. **Beware of portion sizes!** Most restaurant servings are up to three times bigger than recommended. The recommended size of a single serving of meat is about 3–4 ounces, or roughly the size of the palm of your hand or a deck of cards. I know there's no way you can order a 3-ounce piece of meat, so when your dinner arrives, cut the correct portion and take whatever's left home for tomorrow's lunch. Or ask for a half order. Many restaurants are starting to give you this option, especially at lunch.

5. **Steer clear of rich creamy sauces,** which are loaded with fat and calories, and choose those that are tomato-based. Don't be afraid to ask the waiter how each dish is prepared and whether it can be cooked differently. You may feel like Meg Ryan in *When Harry Met Sally,* but you're paying for your meal and you have a right to have it the healthy way you want it. (If a restaurant gives you a hard time, make a note not to go there when you're watching your weight.)

6. **Chicken, fish, and other seafood are usually the healthiest choices** on the menu. Ask to have them baked, broiled, grilled, steamed, poached, or roasted with little oil.

7. **Order an appetizer as your entrée.** I often do this if I'm not feeling overly hungry.

8. **Always ask for the dressing on the side** and then dip the tines of your fork in the dressing before spearing each piece of lettuce. You'll get the salad dressing taste without wasting a lot of calories. Also, balsamic vinegar is a better choice than a creamy ranch dressing.

9. **If your entrée is served with fries, ask for a side of fruit or salad instead.** Let's get real; if your food shows up with fries you're going to eat them.

10. **If you need a little something sweet after your meal, try sorbet, fresh fruit, or sweet herbal tea.** I usually have a few bites of my husband's dessert so I don't feel as though I've missed out. Drink any after-dinner coffee black or with skimmed milk. Cream will put you over the edge.

11. **Watch the alcohol,** especially if you drink before you eat. We tend to lose a little control and end up eating more food. Drink the water on the table!

12. **Eat slowly, chew your food, and eat until you're full, not stuffed.** You're not supposed to feel like you're about to burst after a meal. Listen to your body and your clothes—they will tell you when enough is enough! Most importantly, enjoy your food but keep saying to yourself "everything is fine in moderation."

13. **Don't match your husband, boyfriend, or friends bite for bite.** Men can generally eat more than women can because they have more muscle, and even if your skinny-minnie girlfriend is diving into the nachos or chocolate mousse, she probably ate a lot less during the day or worked out at the gym. Don't get fooled into thinking that if she can do it, you can too.

14. **Avoid all-you-can-eat buffets like the plague.** That huge spread of food is too tempting and will definitely test your willpower. We want to feel like we're getting value for our money—"I paid for it, I'm going to eat it!"

SPECIFIC RESTAURANT TIPS

Chinese: Avoid anything that's coated or deep-fried, such as egg rolls, General Tsao's chicken, sesame chicken, or sweet-and-sour beef. Instead, order stir-fried dishes that contain meat or shrimp with a vegetable

---

MOTIVATION FROM TEAM MALLETT

A simple food scale helped me learn about portion size and totally changed how I prepared my food—especially when I wanted to make something like spaghetti and had no idea what 2 ounces looked like!
—Christine Alfano, 32, Columbia, Maryland

(beef with broccoli or chicken with snow peas) and ask them to make it with a minimal amount of oil (many places will do this). For the lowest-cal entree, fill up on steamed chicken, tofu, or shrimp with the sauce on the side. Chinese soups are also good choices because they're not cream based. Try hot-and-sour or wonton. For rice, go for steamed white or, even better, fiber-rich brown over fried rice.

Japanese: This is my favorite. Sushi is a healthy option because it's low in fat and calories (though some experts don't think kids should eat raw fish). Just make sure to go to a reputable restaurant so the food is fresh, and skip rolls made with mayo (such as spicy tuna) and fried shrimp. Try chicken or salmon teriyaki, steamed (not fried) dumplings, edamame, and broth-based soups such as miso soup. Japanese salads also tend to be low in fat because of their vinegar-based dressings. Bypass tempura dishes, which are high in fat and deep-fried.

Italian: Because restaurant portions of pasta are typically huge, one dish is enough for three people (yes, three!). Dress your pasta with a tomato-based sauce instead of a cream one (such as Alfredo) and don't even look at the fried zucchini or calamari. Trim fat and calories from eggplant or chicken Parmesan by asking them to grill the eggplant or chicken (not bread it). When it comes to pizza, vegetable toppings are healthiest, but if meat is a must-have, just choose one (barbecued chicken is slimmer than pepperoni or sausage) and never order extra cheese. Thin crust tends to have fewer calories than thick, and limit yourself to one or two slices. Round out any Italian meal with a salad and vegetables.

Mexican: Soft-shell tacos are better than hard shells and salsa is lower in calories and fat than guacamole. With fajitas and burritos, choose just one or two toppings such as sour cream, cheese, or guacamole. Or keep low-fat versions of sour cream and shredded cheese in your refrigerator and add them at home. (This way you can monitor how much is being used.) Order regular beans (such as black beans) in place of refried. If you get the taco salad, don't eat the fried shell it comes in and opt for chicken over beef.

Tracey's Tip

Grill veggies to make them more appetizing. Lightly baste them in a tiny bit of olive oil and place them on the grill. Voila—a tasty array of nutritious veggies! Or marinate them in some balsamic vinegar and lightly steam them. I do this all the time so that I can snack on veggies throughout the day.

MENU LANDMINES

Bad Sauce Choices

Alfredo	Butter, cheese, and cream
Bearnaise	White wine, vinegar, egg yolk, and butter
Béchamel	White flour, buttermilk
Carbonara	Bacon, cheese, cream, and whole eggs
Hollandaise	Butter, egg yolk

Healthier Sauce Choices

Any low-calorie or reduction	Vegetable broth or chicken broth
Gazpacho	Tomatoes and veggies with olive oil
Marinara	Tomatoes

Bad Cooking Methods

Au gratin	Fancy name for "with cheese"
Basted	Fat drippings poured over meat
Battered	Coated in fat and flour, and then generally fry in more fat!
Breaded	Breadcrumbs, whole eggs, and butter
Crisp or crispy	Fried in oil
En croûte	Inside a crust

Healthier Cooking Methods

Au jus	Cooked in its own juice (no added oil)
Baked	No oil or butter added to the cooking process; cooked inside an oven
Broiled	Cooked under a high heat
Grilled	Cooked directly over heat
Poached	Cooked in liquid, usually water
Steamed	Cooked over boiling water by the steam

Defuse Food Cravings

1. Wait five minutes for a craving to pass by distracting yourself with other activities (such as taking a walk or doing some household chores).
2. Drink a glass or two of water. This will instantly fill you up on no calories.
3. Choose foods that help increase your sense of fullness—those high in water and rich in fiber—such as fruits and vegetables.

Eat a piece of fruit and a small amount of nut butter or ten almonds. Fruit can also help satisfy a craving for sweets.

4. Slow down when you eat and enjoy every mouthful. This promotes satiety. Realize that it takes your brain twenty minutes to sense that you're full.

Tracey's Tip

Cook a bunch of chicken breasts and steam a bucketload of veggies over the weekend so that you can stock your fridge for the week. This way, ready-made food will be on hand without the hassle of cooking. This is a lifesaver when days get out of control.

MY SUPER FOODS

The following are staples in my kitchen, and you should make them staples in yours too. Fill your pantry and fridge with these goodies and you'll not only get slim but be healthy and reduce your risk of everything from heart disease to cancer.

Turkey is low in fat and high in protein. It's an inexpensive source of iron, zinc, phosphorus, potassium, and B vitamins. Compared with other meats, turkey has fewer calories, less fat, less cholesterol, and very little sodium. One of my family's favorite lunches is a burger made from lean minced turkey meat and whole-grain bread crumbs. Easy to make, low in fat, and super nutritious—team it with cottage cheese and you're in business!

Wild salmon is rich in omega-3 fatty acids, which reduce inflammation and cholesterol. It's also one fish with the lowest amount of mercury, making it a healthy choice to eat at least twice a week. Try making salmon burgers instead of hamburgers for a change. If possible, buy only wild salmon. The farm-raised stuff is injected with additives to give it that pink color and is higher in toxins than wild salmon. I don't know about you, but I don't find eating fish injected with color chemicals appetizing.

Flaxseeds are a good source of essential fatty acids, linoleic acid, B vitamins, iron, zinc, and trace amounts of potassium, magnesium, phosphorus, calcium, vitamin E, and carotene. And they're rich in fiber and protein. One ounce (approximately 4 tablespoons) has about 6 grams of protein and 8 grams of fiber. Buy whole seeds if possible (split ones are exposed to heat, which decreases their nutritional value) and keep them refrigerated. Grind them right before sprinkling them on cereal or adding them to smoothies. Also, don't cook with flaxseed oil. The heat breaks it down, so just add it to food after it's cooked. Another great way to get your fill of flax is in a new bread from Arnold called Natural Flax & Fiber Bread. It's delicious and made without high-fructose corn syrup.

Nuts are not only delicious but also high in calcium, magnesium, and fiber. Walnuts are a good source of omega-3 fatty acids, pecans are rich in vitamin B6 and E, and pine nuts are high in protein. Almonds may slow the sugar rush that occurs after a meal, according to a report in the *Journal of Nutrition*. By inhibiting the release of glucose into the blood after eating, they may minimize the risk of damage to all-important proteins, which the body needs to function and to keep healthy muscle mass. The slower digestion of carbs leads to lower levels of blood insulin, high levels of which inhibit fat burning and cause increased fat storage. By preventing an insulin spike, almonds aid the fat loss process. Researchers conclude that the protective power of almonds comes from the antioxidants they contain. Before eating any high-processed food such as white bread or pasta, eat 1 ounce of almonds to slow the insulin release and keep your sugar levels consistent. Sprinkle almonds and walnuts on your salads, toss pine nuts into a tomato-based sauce, and add peanuts to your smoothies.

> *Tracey's Tip*
>
> Stay away from yogurt-covered fruit and nuts. They often contain more sugar than yogurt and are not as healthy a choice as you may think.

Tea is naturally one of my favorites. As a British gal, I can't go a day without a cup. Thankfully, green and black teas are full of healthy compounds called flavonoids and catechins. Studies have found that some teas may help prevent some cancers, kidney disease, Alzheimer's, osteoporosis, heart disease, high cholesterol, and strokes. One animal study found that green tea not only promotes fat loss but may help with the loss of the flab that accumulates in the tissues lining the abdominal cavity and surrounding the intestines (viscera) and internal organs. The study was performed on mice, but if it worked for them it just might work for us, too. Because tea is an antioxidant, I drink it first thing in the morning about thirty to forty minutes before I work out. I like to think that it's protecting my body from the free radicals it's exposed to during exercise.

Oats are high in fiber, which helps keep you full, and they're said to be good for your heart and even help prevent some cancers. If you have the extra time to cook them, steel-cut oats are the best choice. Rolled oats are still healthy, but often they've been steamed, rolled, resteamed, and toasted. After all this, they lose some of their natural goodness and golden color. Steel-cut oats are whole grains that have been cut into only two or three pieces, so the nutrients and fiber are still intact. They are also high in B-vitamins, calcium, protein, and fiber, containing nearly twice as much fiber as Cream of Wheat. Great for breakfast on a cold winter's day!

Yogurt is creamy, sweet, low in fat and calories, and an amazing source of protein and calcium. Plus, it comes in so many varieties, from squeeze yogurts to drinks, that it's easy to toss in your bag and eat on the go. Some varieties also contain healthy bacteria called lactopacteria and acidophilus, which promote the growth of healthy bacteria in the colon, possibly reducing the risk of cancer. A daily dose of yogurt while taking antibiotics helps replenish the intestines with live bacterial cultures from the yogurt. (Antibiotics kill not only bad bacteria but also the good ones in the intestines.) The best yogurts provide 35–40 percent of the recommended daily allowance of calcium in an 8-ounce container. A good rule of thumb: The higher the protein and the lower the sugar content, the more yogurt in the container. Plain yogurt is more nutritious than flavored yogurt and usually contains more protein and calcium and less sugar or artificial sweeteners. If it's too bland for your sweet tooth, add some berries or dried fruit and mix well. Yummy!

Berries such as strawberries and blueberries are so delicious that they taste like candy. They have so many nutrients there's barely enough room on this page to mention them; these include vitamins A, C, E, and K, beta-carotene, folic acid, potassium, and folate.

DID YOU KNOW?

The USDA has come up with a system for measuring the antioxidant capacity of foods that they call ORAC (oxygen radical absorbance capacity). Fresh blueberries have an ORAC of 2400 per 100 grams. That means 100 grams of these little blue sweet treats could give you as much antioxidants as five servings of some fruits and veggies. Also, researchers specializing in the health benefits of certain plant compounds have found that quercertin, which is plentiful in strawberries, may help destroy cancer cells.

Ounce for ounce, strawberries have more vitamin C than any other citrus fruit. Who knew? And both berries are loaded with antioxidants, among the highest of all fruits and veggies, so they may help ward off diseases such as cancer. Some studies have found that blueberries help with memory function and balance and also reduce cholesterol.

Apples are full of vitamins, which is probably why they say, "An apple a day keeps the doctor away." Some types of apples include calcium, potassium, magnesium, vitamins A and C, beta-carotene, and lutein. Apples also have a high fiber content, which helps prevent constipation and ensure regularity. All that lovely stuff can ward off cancers such as colon cancer.

Citrus fruits such as lemons, limes, oranges, and grapefruits are chock-full of vitamin C, which is believed to boost your immune system and neutralize free radicals. For example, just one orange supplies 116 percent of the daily value for vitamin C. They're also loaded with fiber, calcium, vitamin A, potassium, beta-carotene, folate, and vitamin B5. Plus, pink and red grapefruits contain lycopene, a compound that's known to have cancer-fighting properties.

Avocados are in, so bring on the guacamole! Although they have a high fat content, much of it is the good, monounsaturated kind—such as oleic acid—that may help lower cholesterol. They also contain folic acid, phosphorous, beta-carotene, potassium (more than bananas!), lutein, and vitamins B3, B5, E, and K.

Pomegranates are something I'd never heard of growing up in England. But I'm so glad I discovered them because these babies are nutritional powerhouses. Just one gives you 40 percent of the RDA for vitamin C, and they're also packed with folic acid, calcium, potassium, iron, antioxidants, and compounds known as phytonutrients, which may help protect against heart disease, diabetes, rheumatoid

Tracey's Tip

Make pomegranate juice, an easy, quick, low-calorie, nutritious drink! Place 1 to 1-1/2 cups of seeds in a blender or food processor. Blend until they're liquefied. Pour through a strainer. Refrigerate for up to three days or freeze up to six months. Yields 1 cup of juice. One medium pomegranate (about 9 ounces) yields 1/2 cup juice. One medium pomegranate is about 80 calories.

arthritis, Alzheimer's disease, and cancer. I love drinking Izze Pomegranate, a sparkling drink loaded with juice from this delicious fruit.

Tomatoes are rich in lycopene, a compound that may reduce your risk of heart disease and cancer. One study at the Brigham and Women's Hospital in Boston followed forty thousand women for seven years and found that those who consumed seven to ten servings each week of lycopene-rich foods (tomato-based products, including tomatoes, tomato juice, tomato sauce, and pizza) were found to have a 29 percent lower risk of cardiovascular disease compared to women eating less than 1½ servings of tomato products weekly. An added bonus from eating tomatoes? You get vitamins A, B6, C, and K, and potassium, magnesium, folate, copper, niacin, and iron.

Brassica vegetables is a fancy name for veggies such as broccoli, cabbage, cauliflower, and brussels sprouts. They contain calcium, magnesium, potassium, beta-carotene, folic acid, fiber, and vitamins B6, C, E, and K. Surprisingly, they're also rich in omega-3 fatty acids and protein. Research has shown that this group of veggies may help prevent cancer. In one study of more than three hundred women in Shanghai, China, those who ate the most brassica veggies had a 45 percent lower risk of breast cancer than those who ate the least.

Carrots are not just for bunnies These yummy veggies are an excellent source of antioxidants and have more vitamin A than other vegetables. They're said to help protect against heart disease and cancer and possibly improve your vision. Plus, a bag of baby carrots is a great snack when you want to crunch on something without the calories. Try them dipped in a little hummus or low-fat ranch dressing.

MOTIVATION FROM TEAM MALLETT

*Eating the right blend of foods in small portions throughout the day
really does satisfy my cravings to binge on a bag of chips as well as
provide my body with the fuel to burn fat when doing workouts.*
—*Michelle Eaton, 37, Seattle, Washington*

Asparagus has a reputation for making your pee smell funny. This happens because asparagus stimulates the kidneys and is a natural diuretic, which means asparagus may help when you have a bloated belly during your period or PMS. They're also chock-full of nutrients such as vitamins A, C, K, and B as well as fiber, manganese, copper, phosphorous, and potassium.

Spinach was Popeye's favorite and the guy was on to something. These leafy greens are a great source of vitamins B6, C, A, and K as well as calcium, protein, zinc, fiber, and omega-3 fatty acids. They're said to protect against cancer and they're a great, low-fat way to get iron. "The Environmental Working Group, a consumer advocate and protection nonprofit research organization, put spinach on its list of twelve foods most contaminated with pesticides," says Jonny Bowden, Ph.D., author of *The 150 Healthiest Foods on Earth*. As a result, going organic with this veggie is probably your best bet.

Sweet potatoes should be on your dinner table year-round, not just at Thanksgiving. Bake one and add a dab of butter for a sweet, low-fat, and low-calorie snack or as part of a meal. Do so and you'll get your fill of vitamins A and C, fiber, magnesium, copper, and beta carotene. A study conducted by John Hopkins University researchers linked high levels of beta carotene with a lower incidence of lung cancer.

Quinoa is higher in protein than any other member of the grain family. It has an average of 16.2 percent protein, compared with 7.5 percent for rice, 9.9 percent for millet, and 14 percent for wheat. It is also a good source of dietary fiber, phosphorus, magnesium, and iron.

MOTIVATION FROM TEAM MALLETT

I took the "unlimited vegetables" to the extreme and ate large quantities of raw veggies and felt full all the time. This got me through a tough plateau at four weeks and had me going full throttle again.
—*Tanya Torforson, 28, Bruderheim, Canada*

Success Story

....

Sydney Haughton, 44, Gardner, Massachusetts

Lost

25 pounds

Four dress sizes

2 ½ inches off her arms

4 inches off her waist

3 ½ inches off her hips

4 inches off her legs

14 inches total

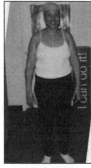

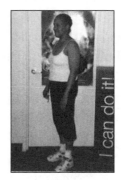

Before   **After**

Gained

A new lease on life and confidence. *Knowing that I can eat healthy and lose weight is so empowering.*

Sydney Haughton, a married mother of two, was ready for a change. A change in her body to be exact. "I was at a reasonable weight for most of my adult life until I had my two kids. After my pregnancies, my weight yo-yoed. It was down one year, up the next," says this night auditor from Gardner, Massachusetts. "The extra weight made me feel thoroughly and absolutely disgusted with myself."

Although she'd tried to slim down on other programs such as L.A. Weight Loss and Weight Watchers and did Tae Bo and walking aerobics, she found Tracey's style and the plan to be a "refreshing change of pace"

SYDNEY'S STICK-WITH-IT TIP

Don't get overwhelmed. Tracey's great wealth of tips and information can be intimidating at first, but you don't have to do everything all at once. Try a couple of changes at a time for a week and then it will be more likely to become a habit.

and loved the workouts. "The exercise program is split up so it is more time efficient and flexible," she says. "I actually like to exercise, but Tracey's program incorporates dance and Pilates moves that I had previously steered clear of."

The hardest part of the program for Sydney was eating healthy on a consistent basis and limiting alcohol. Before joining Team Mallett, her diet was filled with lots of unhealthy, high-fat, and processed foods. Still, Sydney pushed through the tough moments and found that she reaped great results. "Cleaner eating makes for a more efficient and healthier body," she says. "I realized that even small changes could make a difference in my body and health." It's true that thinking small gave Sydney something big. She lost 25 pounds, shops for smaller clothing sizes, and was getting compliments on her slimmer frame from friends and family. "My 7-year-old son even professed that my butt and stomach look much better," she says.

TRACEY'S TAKE

Sydney is learning that exercise and consistency are the keys to a long and healthy life. I know even being showcased in this book has taken a lot of courage on Sydney's behalf. I would like to thank Sydney for letting me into her life and letting me help her. She has proven that she can do it. Look how great she looks. Sydney, continue down the same path of success until you are at a place where you truly feel happy. You're nearly there; don't give up!

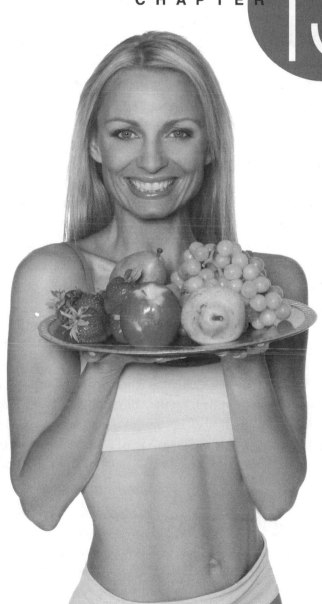

CHAPTER 13

SEXY IN 6
RECIPES

'LL BE THE FIRST TO ADMIT THAT I'M NO RACHAEL RAY OR MARTHA Stewart when it comes to cooking. But I've finally found delicious specialties that I can cook without the smoke alarm going off or without the need for a first aid kit nearby. Okay, I'm exaggerating a bit—I'm not *that* bad.

These recipes are good-for-you meals that have become standbys in my diet—and are so tasty that my husband and kids gladly eat them (little do they know they're dining on healthy fare). To perfect them for you, I worked with Christy Hedges, a well-known chef who graduated from the prestigious California School of Culinary Arts, Le Cordon Bleu. She's also a specialist in nutrition and recipe development and editor-in-chief of a series of textbooks used at the Kitchen Academy, a school that trains professional chefs.

What I love is that these recipes are high in nutrients and antioxidants and they all contain energy-boosting foods that are essential for women. How do I decide whether a delicious recipe is worth it? If I can make it in twenty minutes or less, it goes in my cooking repertoire. Any longer than that and you won't be eating it at my house. All these recipes are a cinch to prepare. Trust me—you'll love 'em!

So now you have no excuse to blow off healthy eating. After all, twenty minutes is quick. It's faster than ordering take-out and much less fattening. And though it's easier to head to a restaurant or fast food place and let someone else do the cooking, the advantages of cooking at home are huge. A new study from the University of Texas found that dieters ate between 200 and 300 extra calories, as well as 10 to 16 extra grams of fat, on days when they dined out. Yikes! Do that just a few times a week for a year and the potential weight gain could be up to 12 pounds!

MOTIVATION FROM TEAM MALLETT

Through the healthy eating plan, I feel like I am fueling my body with better choices. I realize now that in the past I wasn't fueling my body enough. And I am so happy to be eating whole-grain breads again. I had deprived myself of them for years because of what I'd heard about carbs being bad, and now I can enjoy a slice of rye bread, which is my version of heaven!
—Valerie Horrey-Wold, 41, South Pasadena, California

When you eat at home, you choose the ingredients and are in control of the portions. And even when you drive the waiter nuts and ask for no oil or butter on your fish or your chicken grilled dry, the cook may not listen. The bottom line is that eating at home is better for your bottom—and your wallet. It's amazing how much eating out adds up over the course of a month. Do the math. Five lunches a week at about $10 a pop and two dinners a week at $15 a pop comes to a grand conservative cost of $320 a month, and that's just for one person! (Those may be L.A. prices, but even a few bucks less is a wad of cash that's better saved for your kids' college fund or spent on a fabulous pair of shoes!)

WHO KNEW?

Green tea is rich in antioxidants and according to research may boost your immune system and metabolism.

One key tip: Before you get cooking, make sure your kitchen is stocked with all the necessary ingredients for the recipes. I make this easy on myself by going on one big weekly shopping trip and making sure I have staples such as veggies, fruit, brown rice, olive oil, and eggs in the house at all times. Then I make little side trips to pick up fresh produce, seafood, chicken, and so on. So let that pizza and Chinese food delivery guy go to someone else's house. In the meantime, slip on your apron, open the fridge, and get cooking!

BREAKFAST RECIPES

Remember how your mother was always forcing you to eat before you left for school? All I wanted to do was get five more minutes of shut eye, but my mother swore that having breakfast would give me more energy and brain power. Well, Mama, you were right again! Breakfast is the most important meal of the day. You can't blow it off on my plan. Think of this first meal as the light to your furnace, with your furnace being your metabolism.

If you don't eat in the morning, you're bound to be ravenous come noon (or sooner) and make poor food choices such as nibbling that doughnut at the office or zipping through the drive-through for something greasy after taking the kids to school. By eating breakfast, you naturally squeeze in lots of nutrients that are hard to get in at other meals, such as calcium, fiber, and vitamin C, and importantly, you set a healthy tone for the rest of the day. I've included some great breakfast recipes that contain whole-grain fiber to fill you up and keep your energy sustained; some protein to feed your muscles, fuel your metabolism, and boost your immune system; and antioxidant-rich fruit to provide fiber and keep you looking young and beautiful. And don't forget your water! Aim for at least two glasses before you leave the house. My trick is to drink one glass right when I wake up. It makes me feel healthy and energetic.

If you're in a rush try these super-quick, high-energy breakfasts:

1. ½ cup low-fat cottage cheese with chopped strawberries, served on top of 1 piece of whole wheat toast
2. ½ whole-wheat English muffin topped with 1 ounce of part-skim ricotta cheese and 1 slice of Canadian bacon
3. 1 whole-grain frozen waffle topped with ½ cup low-fat cottage cheese
4. ½ cup cooked quick oatmeal mix, 1 scoop of protein whey powder, and 1 tablespoon of flaxseed, topped with blueberries

The rest of the time, try these easy morning meals.

MOTIVATION FROM TEAM MALLETT

Everyone knows that sensible eating and exercise are the key to healthful living, but the trouble is in the details. Tracey's program tells you how to move toward that goal. I know so many people who go on horrible diets only to feel so deprived that they abandon them before they lose the weight. In their state of deprivation, they end up eating all the foods they missed and often gain more weight than they lost. Tracey's program is balanced, offers good food, and gets the weight off with exercise. You don't feel hungry and you know that you are getting stronger.
—Suanne Mendell, 60, La Canada, California

SEXY IN 6 RECIPES • 263

FOOD EXCHANGES

BERRY PROTEIN SMOOTHIE

FOOD EXCHANGE: 2 FRUIT, 2 PROTEIN, 1/2 DAIRY, 1 FAT
Serving size: One

1 cup frozen blueberries or strawberries (berries are powerhouse
    sources of antioxidants)
⅓ cup pomegranate juice (pomegranates may slow aging and fight heart
    disease)
½ cup of light soy milk
1 scoop (15 grams) whey powder (a great source of protein)
¼ teaspoon ground cinnamon (helps regulate blood sugar levels)
1 tablespoon freshly ground flaxseeds (an excellent source of omega-3
    and fiber that helps to suppress hunger)

Place all ingredients in a blender and blend on high for one minute.

PAPAYA PINEAPPLE PROTEIN SMOOTHIE

FOOD EXCHANGE: 2-1/2 FRUIT, 2 PROTEIN, 1 FAT

½ ripe papaya (good for digestion and is an anti-inflammatory)
½ cup fresh or frozen pineapple (also good for digestion)
½ cup frozen strawberries
1 cup coconut water (not coconut milk)
1 scoop (15 grams) whey powder
1 tablespoon freshly ground flaxseeds

Place all ingredients in a blender and blend on high for one minute.

BANANA SMOOTHIE

FOOD EXCHANGE: 1-1/2 FRUIT, 1 PROTEIN, 1 DAIRY, 1 FAT
Serving size: One

1 small banana (a good source of potassium and fiber)
½ cup frozen strawberries
½ teaspoon vanilla extract
1 cup vanilla soy milk (low-fat soy milk or non-fat)
1 tablespoon almond butter

Place all ingredients in a blender and blend on high for one minute.

VEGETABLE OMELET

FOOD EXCHANGE: 1-1/2 PROTEIN, 1 DAIRY, 1 GRAIN, 5 VEGETABLE,
1 FAT IF NOT COOKED WITH SPRAY
Serving size: One
Serving suggestion: Serve with ½ whole-wheat English muffin

1 teaspoon olive oil or non-fat olive oil spray
1 cup broccoli florets, chopped
½ cup chopped tomatoes
½ cup sliced button or cremini mushrooms
½ cup chopped green bell pepper
3 egg whites, beaten
½ cup shredded reduced-fat cheddar or Monterey Jack cheese

Preheat an 8-inch nonstick sauté pan and add the olive oil. Once the oil is hot, add the vegetables and sauté over medium heat until tender. Remove the vegetables from the pan and set aside. Spray the pan with a small amount of olive oil only if needed and pour in the beaten egg whites. Tilt the pan and cook the egg whites briefly until slightly set. Add the reserved vegetables to the center of the egg whites. Continue to cook the eggs until done. Fold the omelet in half over the vegetables and serve.

OATMEAL WITH BLUEBERRIES AND WALNUTS

FOOD EXCHANGE: 2 GRAIN, 1/2 DAIRY, 1 FRUIT, 1FAT
Serving size: One

½ cup uncooked oatmeal (steel cut if possible; an excellent low-gluten whole grain)
½ cup low-fat milk or soy milk
½ cup blueberries
¼ cup roasted walnuts

Cook oatmeal. Add blueberries and stir to combine. Serve with milk and sprinkled with walnuts.

POACHED EGG ON TOAST

FOOD EXCHANGE: 1 PROTEIN, 1 GRAIN, 2 VEGETABLE 1 FRUIT
Serving size: One
Serving suggestion: Serve with a piece of fruit

1 egg
1 piece of whole-grain toast
1 cup cooked and drained spinach (an excellent source of lutein, which is good for vision)
2 tablespoons salsa

Poach an egg in a pot of hot water. Remove and drain well. Place the toast in the middle of a plate, place the spinach on top, and then nestle the egg on top of the spinach. Top with salsa.

WHO KNEW?

Studies show that eating out of large packages and containers can lead to overeating—even if we don't like what we're munching on. Researchers at Cornell Food and Brand Lab at Cornell University gave moviegoers 8-ounce or 4-ounce tubs of stale, fourteen-day-old popcorn. Those who watched the flick with their giant-sized buckets ate 34 percent more than those who got the smaller portions. And the popcorn was stale! In fact, moviegoers described it as "terrible," but they still nibbled away.

WAFFLE BREAKFAST

FOOD EXCHANGE: 1 GRAIN, 1/2 DAIRY, 1/2 FRUIT
Serving size: One

1 frozen whole-wheat waffle
½ cup low-fat Greek yogurt
1 teaspoon honey
½ cup sliced strawberries

Cook the waffle according to the directions on the package. In a small bowl, whip together the yogurt and the honey. Serve on top of the waffle. Top with the sliced strawberries.

SALMON FRITTATA

FOOD EXCHANGE: 4-1/2 PROTEIN, 1 FAT, PLUS 1 MORE FAT IF NOT COOKED WITH SPRAY
Serving size: One

Nonfat olive oil spray
3 egg whites
1 egg
1 teaspoon low-fat milk
1 teaspoon chopped fresh dill
Pinch of salt
Pinch of pepper
2 ounces smoked salmon or lox that is not too salty, diced
¼ cup of low-fat cream cheese or Neufchâtel
1 teaspoon low-fat sour cream

Preheat oven to 400° F. Heat an 8-inch skillet or omelet pan. Spray pan with olive oil spray or lightly coat with a small amount of olive oil. In a medium bowl, beat together egg whites, egg, milk, dill, and a pinch of salt and pepper. Stir in the smoked salmon and the low-fat cream cheese or

Neufchâtel. Pour mixture into the skillet. Cook lightly until the eggs are set only on the bottom; the center should still be wet. Transfer the skillet to the oven and cook until the eggs are set and slightly puffy. This should take about five minutes. Serve with a spoonful of low-fat sour cream.

WHO KNEW?

Researchers at Cornell University found that using a short glass can make you pour 20 to 30 percent more of a beverage into that glass. As a result, this may mean you'll drink more. This is not a good thing if what you're sipping is alcohol or a calorie-laden beverage such as soda or juice. But if you're trying to boost your intake of water or unsweetened ice tea, go short.

LUNCH RECIPES

My lunch choices include foods that will satisfy your midday hunger and keep you feeling strong all day. Team Mallett had a common goal: They all wanted to increase their energy and stop the midafternoon crash. And they're not alone. This is a major problem for women, especially when they're on the go (and who isn't these days?). But when you're running around all the time, it's easy to not eat and then make bad decisions in a race to get food down before you collapse. Sound familiar? Eating a well-balanced lunch that combines protein, fiber, and fruit will keep you full and your metabolism running smoothly. Another perk of protein: Your body uses it on a regular basis throughout the day to repair muscles and build your new beautiful physique.

WHO KNEW?

Get that broccoli cooking. New research suggests that as little as a daily serving or two of brassica vegetables—a fancy word for those like broccoli, cauliflower, and Brussels sprouts—may decrease your risk of cancer by blocking production of free radicals.

TUNA SALAD SERVED IN A TOMATO

FOOD EXCHANGE: 3 PROTEIN, 1 VEGETABLE, 1 GRAIN, 1/2 FAT
Serving size: One
Serving suggestion: Serve with two whole-grain crackers or a piece of whole-grain bread

½ 6-ounce can of water-packed tuna
1 teaspoon minced green onion
1 teaspoon lemon juice
1 teaspoon low-fat mayonnaise
1 medium large tomato (a good source of lycopene, which helps fight cancer)

Mix together all ingredients, except the tomato, and set aside. Cut the top off the tomato and hollow out the seeds and the middle section. Fill the tomato with the tuna mixture.

MOTIVATION FROM TEAM MALLETT

By eating the foods Tracey recommends, I don't feel hungry and don't crave sweets like I used to. I'm usually an emotional eater and even during a very stressful month for me I didn't eat out of stress. Plus, I've lost my taste for sweets. I had a doughnut during the fourth week and had a headache the whole day!
—Kim Sinclair, 46, Alhambra, Los Angeles

SPINACH SALAD WITH LEMON YOGURT DRESSING

FOOD EXCHANGE: 2 DAIRY, 5 VEGETABLE, 2 GRAIN, 2 FAT

Serving size: One

Serving suggestion: Serve with one 6-inch wheat pita bread

2 cups baby spinach (an excellent source of folic acid, good for heart
and brain health)

½ cup of green onions, chopped

½ cup cucumber, chopped

6 cherry tomatoes cut in half

2 ounces feta cheese, crumbled

¼ cup toasted walnuts (have the highest amount of omega-3s of any nut)

Dressing:

1 tablespoon low-fat Greek yogurt

½ teaspoon water

1 teaspoon olive oil

½ teaspoon fresh lemon juice

¼ teaspoon garlic powder

Pinch dried oregano

Salt and pepper to taste

Toss all the salad ingredients in a bowl. In a separate small bowl, whisk
together the yogurt, water, olive oil, lemon juice, garlic powder, oregano,
and salt and pepper. Pour the dressing over the salad and toss well to
coat all ingredients.

BLACK BEAN SOUP

FOOD EXCHANGE: 1 PROTEIN, 3 GRAIN, 1 FAT, 1 VEGETABLE
(FOOD EXCHANGE PER SERVING FOR ONE PERSON)
Serving size: Two
Serving suggestion: Serve the soup with half a 6-inch whole grain pita

2 cups of black beans, rinsed and drained (a great source of fiber)
2 teaspoons olive oil
½ cup of onion, chopped
1 clove garlic, minced
½ cup of celery, chopped
½ cup of carrot, chopped
Pinch of red pepper flakes
1 cup low-salt chicken stock
1 teaspoon Worcestershire sauce
Dash of hot sauce

Garnish:
1 hard-boiled egg, sliced

Rinse beans and set aside to drain. Heat the olive oil in a small, heavy-bottomed pot. Add the onion, garlic, celery, carrot, and red pepper flakes and sauté over medium heat until the onion is translucent and the vegetables are tender. Add the beans, chicken stock, and Worcestershire sauce and simmer for ten to twenty minutes. When done, place the contents in a blender with the top on tight. Cover with a tea towel in case the hot liquid splatters and blend on a low speed until smooth. Adjust thickness as necessary with additional chicken stock. Taste for salt and pepper, and add a dash of hot sauce if desired. Serve 1 cup of the soup with a half a sliced hard-boiled egg on top.

CAESAR SALAD WITH SHRIMP OR CHICKEN

FOOD EXCHANGE: 4 PROTEIN, 1 DAIRY, 1/2 GRAIN, 2 VEGETABLE, 1 FAT

4 ounces cooked, peeled medium shrimp or cooked chicken tenders cut
   into strips
2 cups romaine lettuce, chopped
1 ounce shaved parmesan cheese
½ cup whole-wheat baked croutons

Dressing:
½ clove garlic, minced
1 teaspoon lemon juice
1 teaspoon reduced-fat mayonnaise
½ teaspoon Dijon mustard
⅛ teaspoon freshly ground pepper
⅛ teaspoon salt
1 teaspoon water
1 teaspoon olive oil

  In a small bowl, mix together all ingredients for the dressing except the olive oil. Then slowly drizzle in the olive oil, whisking constantly. Toss the shrimp or chicken, lettuce leaves, and croutons with the dressing. Serve the shaved parmesan on top of the salad.

TURKEY BURGER WITH RANCH DRESSING

FOOD EXCHANGE: 4 PROTEIN, 1 DAIRY, 2 GRAIN, 1/2 VEGETABLE, 1 FRUIT
(FOOD EXCHANGE PER SERVING FOR ONE PERSON)
Serving size: Makes four 4-ounce patties
Serving suggestion: Serve each portion with an apple cut into wedges
and sprinkled with cinnamon

1 pound (16 ounces) fresh ground turkey meat
2 egg whites, lightly beaten
¼ cup whole-grain breadcrumbs (such as Ezekiel bread)
1 tablespoon Dijon mustard
1 teaspoon dried thyme
1 teaspoon dried oregano
½ teaspoon garlic powder
⅛ teaspoon cayenne pepper
¼ teaspoon salt

In a medium-sized bowl, mix together all the ingredients. Divide the
mixture into four equal parts and form each portion into a patty. These
patties may be cooked immediately or frozen to use later.

1 4-ounce turkey burger
1 slice reduced-fat cheese
2 slices or ½ cup of tomato
1 romaine lettuce leaf
1 whole-wheat bun

Dressing:
1 teaspoon reduced-fat mayonnaise
1 teaspoon low-fat Greek yogurt
⅛ teaspoon garlic powder
1 teaspoon chopped chives
1 teaspoon chopped green onion
Pinch of salt
Pinch of pepper

Heat a skillet over medium heat and spray with cooking spray. Cook the turkey burger until almost done. Add the slice of cheese on top and cover with a lid until the cheese has melted. Toast the whole-wheat bun. Whisk together all ingredients for the dressing in a small bowl. Place the turkey burger on top of the bun and spread with the dressing. Add the tomato and lettuce.

CHICKEN PITA PIZZA

FOOD EXCHANGE: 2 PROTEIN, 2 DAIRY, 2 GRAIN, 1 VEGETABLE
Serving size: One

1 6-inch whole-wheat pita
¼ cup marinara sauce—look for one without sugar (the lycopene in cooked tomatoes is more available than in raw tomatoes)
2 ounces sliced, cooked low-fat Italian turkey sausage (about ½ sausage)
½ cup (2–3) button or cremini mushrooms, thinly sliced
½ cup shredded, part-skim mozzarella cheese

Preheat the oven to 500°F. Place the pita on a baking sheet and heat briefly on a center rack in the oven, about two to three minutes. Remove from the oven and brush with marinara sauce. Distribute sausage and mushroom slices on top of the sauce and sprinkle with the cheese. Place the pan back in the oven until the sauce is hot and the cheese is bubbling, about five minutes.

REFRIED BEAN TOSTADA

FOOD EXCHANGE: 2 GRAIN, 2 DAIRY, 2-1/2 VEGETABLE
Serving size: One

1 6-inch whole-grain tortilla
½ cup no-fat or low-fat vegetarian refried beans
¼ cup chopped green onion
½ cup shredded part-skim mozzarella or reduced-fat Monterey Jack
  cheese
2 cups of Romaine or iceberg lettuce, shredded
½ cup of tomato, chopped
¼ cup salsa

Preheat the oven to 350°F. Place the tortilla on a baking sheet and heat for one to two minutes. Remove from the oven and spread the refried beans on top of the tortilla. Sprinkle with the green onion, tomato, and cheese. Place in the oven until hot, about five to six minutes. Top with lettuce and salsa.

DINNER RECIPES

Yea! It's time to sit, relax, and enjoy dinner. If that sounds like something impossible with your family's hectic schedule, consider this. Research shows that kids who eat with their parents several times a week are less likely to get involved in drugs and alcohol. Eating dinner together is also enjoyable and something great to look forward to during a busy, stressful day. I know it's not easy to do nightly, but shoot for a few times a week.

Meals don't have to be elaborate, which is one reason you'll love these dinner recipes. You can make them quickly. In general, try not to eat dinner too late; instead, give your body enough time to digest the food before going to bed. Limit your grains to one or two servings because you need the energy they provide more throughout the day, rather than when you're going to hit the sack. Enjoy these quick, easy dinners and watch your energy soar tomorrow!

SEARED SEA SCALLOPS

FOOD EXCHANGE: 4 PROTEIN, 1 FAT, 1 GRAIN

Serving size: One

Serving suggestion: Serve with ½-cup quinoa or brown rice (quinoa is actually a highly nutritious seed but is used like a grain and is high in protein)

4 ounces sea scallops (look for "dry" scallops that have not been injected with chemicals to artificially plump them, because they will not brown as well)

1 teaspoon macadamia nut oil (macadamia oil is rich in heart-healthy oleic acid)

Freshly ground black pepper

Sauce:

1 teaspoon grated fresh ginger

1 teaspoon low sodium soy sauce

1 teaspoon fresh lime juice

Preheat an iron skillet. Add the macadamia nut oil. After the oil is very hot, add the scallops (being careful not to crowd). As soon as the scallops are nicely browned and will easily release from the bottom of the pan, turn them over, and sear the other side in the same way. Be careful not to overcook. Remove from the pan and drain away any excess oil.

Whisk together the ginger, soy sauce, and lime juice. Serve the scallops on top of the quinoa or brown rice and pour the sauce over the top.

Tracey's Tip

If the oil is hot in a sauté pan before adding other ingredients, much less of the oil is absorbed into the food. Instead, it remains in the pan and is necessary only to keep the food from sticking during cooking.

ASIAN COLE SLAW

FOOD EXCHANGE: 3-1/2 VEGETABLE, 1 FAT
Serving size: One
Serving suggestion: Try this side dish with the preceding recipe,
Seared Sea Scallops

1 cup shredded green cabbage
1 cup shredded red cabbage
1 cup or large carrot, grated
½ to 1 green onion, minced
1 teaspoon toasted sesame seeds

Dressing:
1 tablespoon seasoned rice vinegar
1 teaspoon olive oil

Toss the cabbage, carrot, green onion, and sesame seeds together. Whisk
the rice vinegar and olive oil together and pour over the cabbage mixture.

VEGETABLE AND TOFU STIR FRY

FOOD EXCHANGE: 1 PROTEIN, 1 GRAIN, 2 VEGETABLE, 2 FAT
Serving size: One
Serving suggestion: Serve over ½ cup brown rice

½ cup of firm tofu (retains its shape when cooked)
2 cups sliced vegetables (choose from any combination: broccoli,
    onions, red bell peppers, snap peas, mushrooms, bean sprouts)
2 teaspoons macadamia nut oil

Sauce:
1 tablespoon low-sodium soy sauce
1 teaspoon mirin (Japanese cooking wine)
1 teaspoon grated fresh ginger (boosts the immune system and aids
    in digestion)
¼ teaspoon sesame oil

Weight a cake of tofu (with a heavy skillet or something similar) for about ten minutes, then place on paper towels to drain. Cut the tofu into 1-inch cubes. Combine sauce ingredients in a small bowl and whisk together.

Use a small, flat, nonstick skillet (so that the vegetables will cook evenly). Preheat a nonstick sauté pan and add the oil. Add the broccoli, onions, and peppers first, and then add the snap peas, mushrooms, and bean sprouts. Cook until tender, but still crisp. Add the tofu and continue to cook until the tofu is hot. Whisk together the ingredients for the sauce and pour over the tofu and vegetables. Gently stir, being careful not to break the tofu.

BROCCOLI CHEESE FRITTATA

FOOD EXCHANGE: 2-1/2 PROTEIN, 2 DAIRY, 1-1/2 VEGETABLE
Serving size: One
Serving suggestion: Serve with a green salad dressed with olive oil and
seasoned rice vinegar dressing, or serve with Asian Cole Slaw.

Nonfat olive oil spray
2 tablespoons chopped onions
1 clove garlic, chopped
¼ cup chopped red bell pepper
½ cup chopped broccoli
½ cup chopped Roma tomato
¼ teaspoon fresh basil, chopped
1 whole egg
3 egg whites
Salt and pepper, to taste
Pinch red pepper flakes
½ cup shredded part-skim mozzarella or reduced fat Monterey Jack
    cheese

Preheat the oven to 350°F. Heat an 8-inch nonstick pan with the olive oil
spray. Sauté onions, garlic, bell pepper, and broccoli over low heat until
the onions are translucent and the vegetables are tender. Add tomatoes
and basil and stir. Beat the eggs together with the salt and pepper and
pour over the vegetables. Stir briefly and cook just until sides are set,
about two to three minutes. Sprinkle cheese on top and put the pan in
the oven for about three minutes, or until the frittata gets puffy and the
eggs are set but still moist.

VEGETARIAN CHILI

FOOD EXCHANGE: 1-1/2 VEGETABLE, 3 GRAIN, PLUS 1 FAT (DELETE FAT IF
COOKING WITH NONFAT OLIVE OIL SPRAY)
(FOOD EXCHANGE PER SERVING FOR ONE PERSON)
Serving size: Two
Serving suggestion: Serve with one 6-inch whole-grain tortilla per
person

2 cups of cooked pinto beans
2 teaspoons olive oil or nonfat olive oil spray
½ cup of chopped onion
1 clove garlic, minced
1–2 teaspoons chile powder
1 teaspoon dried oregano leaves
1 teaspoon dried cumin powder
½ cup canned crushed tomatoes
2 ounces or ½ cup canned chopped green chilies, drained
1 cup vegetable stock, as needed
Salt and pepper to taste

Garnish:
1 teaspoon low-fat sour cream
1 teaspoon chopped green onions
Hot sauce

Rinse beans and set aside to drain. Heat the oil in a small pot and add the
onions and garlic. Sauté over low heat until the onions are translucent
and soft. Add the chile powder, oregano, and cumin. Stir and cook for
about two minutes, being careful not to burn the mixture. Add the tomatoes, chilies, and beans. Simmer for ten to twenty minutes. Add the vegetable stock; bring the mixture to a boil and lower to a simmer. Put a lid
on the pot and simmer for about twenty minutes until the mixture is a
nice consistency. Salt and pepper to taste. Garnish the chili with low-fat
sour cream, chopped green onions, and hot sauce if desired.

ORANGE AND JICAMA SALAD

FOOD EXCHANGE: 1/2 FRUIT, 1 GRAIN, 1 FAT
Serving size: One
Serving suggestion: Serve this side dish with Vegetarian Chili

½ cup sliced jicama
½ orange, sectioned
1 cup butter lettuce

Dressing:
1 teaspoon lime juice
1 teaspoon orange juice
1 teaspoon olive oil
1 teaspoon chopped fresh cilantro
Pinch of salt
Pinch of pepper

Arrange several lettuce leaves on a plate and top with the jicama and orange sections. Mix the dressing ingredients together. Drizzle the dressing over the top of the salad.

MOTIVATION FROM TEAM MALLETT

I love the jicama orange salad. I recently discovered jicama and have been looking for things to do with it other than just slice it up and eat it plain. I took a bowl of the salad to work and it was gone in no time.
—Tanya Torforson, 28, Bruderheim, Canada

POACHED SALMON

FOOD EXCHANGE: 4 PROTEIN, 2 VEGETABLE, 1 GRAIN
Serving size: One
Serving suggestion: Serve with 1 small potato and a green salad

1 4-ounce wild Alaskan salmon fillet (red salmon is one of the best
    sources of omega-3s, which are beneficial for the heart and brain)
¼ teaspoon dried oregano leaves
Salt and pepper, as desired
1½ cups small carrot, sliced
¼ small onion, sliced
¼ stalk celery, sliced
1 slice lemon
Sprig parsley
½ bay leaf
½ cup vegetable stock
1 tablespoon fresh lemon juice

Rub the salmon with the dried oregano leaves and salt and pepper. Place
the salmon fillet in a small nonstick sauté pan. Add the vegetables,
lemon, parsley, and bay leaf on top of the salmon. Gently pour the stock
and lemon juice over the top. Bring the liquid to a boil and immediately
turn down to a simmer. Cover the pan and continue to simmer for about
five minutes. Turn off the heat and allow the fish to steep in the liquid
with the lid on for about eight to ten minutes, or until the fish is cooked
to the desired doneness.

BROILED STEAK SALAD

FOOD EXCHANGE: 4 PROTEIN, 4 VEGETABLE, 1 FAT
Serving size: One

1 4-ounce filet mignon, trimmed of fat
Salt and pepper
2 cups arugula (loaded with minerals and antioxidants and helps protect
    against toxins)
½ cup red bell pepper, cut into ½-inch strips
3 green onions, trimmed
1 cup or 5 stalks asparagus, trimmed
Olive oil, just enough to brush over vegetables

Dressing:
1 teaspoon low-sodium soy sauce
½ teaspoon sesame oil
2 teaspoons seasoned rice vinegar
½ teaspoon grated fresh ginger
⅛ teaspoon garlic powder
Pinch red pepper flakes

Preheat the broiler. Whisk together the dressing ingredients and set aside. Sprinkle the steak with salt and pepper. Brush the red bell pepper, green onions, and asparagus with a very small amount of olive oil. Place the steak on a broiler pan along with the vegetables and place under the broiler. Broil for about three to four minutes. Turn the steak and vegetables over and continue to broil for about another three to four minutes until the steak is done and the vegetables are slightly charred. Set the steak aside on a cutting board for about five minutes. Cut the green onions and asparagus into ½-inch pieces. Toss the arugula and all the broiled vegetables with the dressing. Slice the steak and serve on top of the salad.

CHICKEN FAJITAS

FOOD EXCHANGE: 4 PROTEIN, 1-1/2 VEGETABLE, 1 GRAIN, PLUS 1 FAT
(DELETE FAT IF COOKING WITH NONFAT OLIVE OIL SPRAY)
Serving size: One

4 ounces chicken tenders, sliced into ½-inch strips
½ green bell pepper, sliced into ½-inch strips
½ red bell pepper, sliced into ½-inch strips
½ red onion, sliced
¼ cup lime juice
1 teaspoon ground cumin
¼ teaspoon salt
Pinch cayenne pepper
1 teaspoon of olive oil or nonfat olive oil spray
pinch of black pepper
1 whole-grain 6-inch tortilla

Garnish:
1 teaspoon chopped fresh cilantro
1 tablespoon reduced-fat sour cream

In a medium bowl, mix together the chicken strips, bell peppers, and onion. In another small bowl, whisk together the lime juice, cumin, salt, pepper, and cayenne, and pour over the chicken-and-vegetable mixture. Marinate for ten minutes. Coat a nonstick skillet with cooking spray and heat over medium-high heat. Add the chicken and vegetables to the skillet and sauté over medium heat until done. Serve with whole-grain tortilla and a garnish of sour cream and cilantro.

CHICKEN AND VEGETABLE SOUP

FOOD EXCHANGE: 2 PROTEIN, 1 VEGETABLE, 1/2 GRAIN
(FOOD EXCHANGE PER SERVING FOR ONE PERSON)
Serving size: Four
Serving suggestion: Serve with a small green salad dressed with olive oil and rice vinegar or a low-fat vinaigrette dressing

4 cups low-sodium chicken stock
8 ounces of boneless chicken breasts or 2 skinless chicken breasts, cut into 1-inch pieces
1 cup of onion, diced
1 cup of carrots, cut into 1-inch slices
1 celery stalk with leaves, cut into 1-inch slices
2 potatoes or sweet potatoes, cut into 1-inch chunks
2 cups baby spinach
½ teaspoon dried oregano
4 sprigs fresh parsley
1 teaspoon fresh lemon juice
salt and pepper to taste

Combine stock, chicken, and onions in a covered pot and bring to a boil over medium-high heat. As soon as the mixture reaches a boil, remove the cover and lower the heat to a simmer. Add carrots, celery, potato, baby spinach, oregano, and parsley. Cover the pot again and simmer until the vegetables are tender. Add the lemon juice and salt and pepper to taste. Remove the parsley sprigs before serving.

DESSERT RECIPES

Yes, you read that correctly. It does say "Dessert" because a healthy eating plan can, and in fact should, include some sweet treats. It's unrealistic to expect you to live the rest of your life without them. And if you banish dessert from your life forever, you'll feel deprived and probably wind up bingeing on it at some point anyway. Include dessert in your plan and it won't have such power over you.

Just choose your indulgences wisely. Lots of times I'm satisfied with a nice cup of after-dinner herbal tea and a piece of juicy, fresh fruit or one or two individually wrapped pieces of chocolate (Hershey's Kisses are a favorite of mine and Team Mallett). But when I need a little more, here are a few of my favorites that are low in calories. Your sweet tooth will thank me!

MANGO WHIP

FOOD EXCHANGE: 1/2 DAIRY, 1 FRUIT, 1/2 FAT
(FOOD EXCHANGE PER SERVING FOR ONE PERSON)
Serving size: Two

1 container (5½ ounces) nonfat Greek yogurt
1 ripe mango, pureed
1 tablespoon unsweetened shredded coconut, toasted
2 teaspoons minced crystallized ginger

Whip together the yogurt and mango puree and then divide it between two dessert glasses. Sprinkle the coconut and ginger on top.

WHO KNEW?

A study at the Plant Research International Center in the Netherlands found that raspberries may have ten times more cancer-fighting antioxidants than tomatoes or broccoli, veggies with reputations as potent sources of antioxidants. Plus, these little red fruits may contain a rare type of antioxidant.

STRAWBERRY REFRESHER

FOOD EXCHANGE: 1 FRUIT
Serving size: One

1 cup sliced strawberries
½ teaspoon honey
½ teaspoon lemon juice
1 tablespoon chopped basil

Mix together the strawberries, honey, lemon juice, and basil. Serve in a dessert glass.

BANANA COCOA TREAT

FOOD EXCHANGE: 2 FRUIT, 1 FAT
Serving size: One

1 banana, sliced
¼ teaspoon pure vanilla extract
1 teaspoon apple juice

Garnish
Cinnamon
Unsweetened cocoa powder
5 roasted unsalted almonds, chopped

Mix together the banana, vanilla, and apple juice. Serve in a dessert glass and sprinkle with cocoa, cinnamon, and almonds.

PINEAPPLE MANGO FRUIT SALAD

FOOD EXCHANGE: 2 FRUIT

Serving size: One

⅓ cup chopped fresh pineapple
⅓ cup chopped mango
¼ teaspoon pure vanilla extract
1 teaspoon orange juice
1 teaspoon chopped mint

Mix together the pineapple, mango, vanilla extract, orange juice, and mint. Serve in a dessert glass.

Success Story

· ·

Valerie Horrey-Wold, 41, South Pasadena, California

Lost

6 pounds
4 percent body fat
One dress size
1 inch off her waist
2 inches off her hips
1½ inches off her chest
2 inches off her thighs
6½ inches total

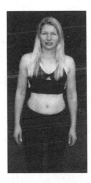

Before

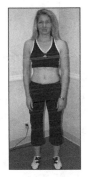

After

Gained

A healthy future. *My mother is recovering from a catastrophic illness, which left her completely paralyzed. Through her life-changing crisis, I learned that the healthier and stronger I am, the more resilient I will be if I* *ever face a serious illness. I see this new lifestyle as an investment into my healthy future.*

• • • • •

In her teens and twenties, Valerie Horrey-Wold, 41, was one of those lucky women the rest of us love to hate. She could eat whatever she wanted, never exercise, and not gain an ounce. All that came to an end in her 30s, and by age 40, what she calls "the extra pudge" wouldn't budge. "I was very self-conscious and unhappy with my body," says this elementary-school teacher. "Over the past six years, I'd slowly gained weight and it seemed like any muscles I had were replaced by fat! I couldn't fit into my clothes anymore, but shopping for larger sizes depressed me. I hated wearing jeans or putting on a bathing suit."

Although Valerie knew Tracey from her studio and knew what fabulous shape Tracey was in, she was skeptical when she heard about *Sexy in 6*. "I'd been working out at the gym five to six days a week for two hours with little results, so I wasn't convinced that six-minute spurts and cardio three times a week would be enough to help me drop the weight," she says. Valerie was stunned when she saw results after just two weeks. She loved how the workouts could be broken up throughout the day and that they were brief while working several muscle groups at a time. "It's a very efficient way to work out and get results. On really busy days, I still have no excuse not to squeeze in a quick blast," she says. "And even when I'm tired and don't feel like exercising, it's easier to motivate myself knowing that it's only going to be a short period of hard work, not a long drawn-out workout." Today, Valerie actually plans her day around her exercise time.

Another shocker was how bad her so-called "healthy" no-carb diet was. "I realized that I was starving myself and had thrown my body into fat-storing mode," she recalls. "I wasn't fueling up enough or at the right

VALERIE'S STICK-WITH-IT TIP

Don't leave home without a snack. Always take food with you whenever you leave the house. This way, you're not caught starving, off-guard, and ready to grab anything in sight!

times." Learning about portion control and eating small meals to keep your metabolism humming along changed all this. "I no longer have cravings or temptations to binge," she says. "And I'm so happy to be eating carbs—like rye bread and fruit—again." The plan also fit easily into Valerie's life. "It doesn't require unusual ingredients, just simply shopping on the perimeter of the grocery store," she says. "It's also easy to stick to because it doesn't eliminate any food groups so I never felt deprived or really hungry."

Others noticed the changes in Valerie's appearance early on. Her coworkers commented on her flat abs, her sister was surprised by how solid Valerie felt when she hugged her, and her husband said she looked hot! More importantly, Valerie now loves herself more and her body image has received a huge boost. "I feel more positive about myself and more motivated to continue to improve my physical fitness," she says. "Which way to the beach?"

TRACEY'S TAKE

Valerie was already quite small to start with after losing 10 pounds as a result of the stress from her mother's illness. But those last 5–8 pounds are the most stubborn to lose—especially when they're around your midsection and you're in your 40s—and Valerie did it with determination. To make the gains in her body that she did in the short period of six weeks was a major accomplishment. Watching her mother fight to walk again put her life in perspective. If her mom could make it to the gym to learn to walk again, Valerie felt she had no excuse. Now, she has a gorgeous, lean body that even a model would envy. Who would have thought that she could look better in her 40s than in her 30s? Look at her. It's possible!

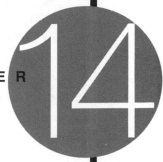

CHAPTER 14

SEXY IN 6
MOTIVATION
JOURNAL

'M A BIG FAN OF WRITING THINGS DOWN. AS YOU KNOW, I THINK writing down what you eat is a good way to stay honest about what you pop in your mouth. I also think writing down your thoughts each week is a good idea. First, it gets these emotions out of your head and on paper—and by some magic that helps you sort things out, see them more clearly, and stop dwelling on them. Second, recording your thoughts can lift you up and spur you on when your motivation is lagging. After all, if you flip back and read about how amazing you felt after a fabulous run or a great week of healthy eating, you'll be reminded of that feeling and inspired to keep up the good work.

The last reason I like recording thoughts is because it will show you how far you've come and remind you to give yourself a well-deserved pat on the back. As women, we're big on handing out praise to everyone from our children to our siblings to the FedEx guy when he arrives on time. But we never stop our go-go-go lives to look ourselves in the mirror and say, "I'm proud of you." So use this journal to jot down your thoughts. You'll be amazed and full of pride when you read it in the weeks to come.

Tracey's Tip

Always try to be optimistic. You will experience ups and downs, but ride them with a smile and stay focused. Every day is a learning experience, and going through the low times makes us truly appreciate the highs.

TEAM MALLETT'S TAKE

I'm very excited and motivated to have something to follow. I have tried everything out there other than having a gastric bypass, which I refuse to do. I know I can do this if I put my heart, mind, and soul into it. I want to be around a long time for my two young children and my husband.
—Randi Hsu, 41, Short Hills, New Jersey

JOURNAL MOTIVATION FOR EACH WEEK

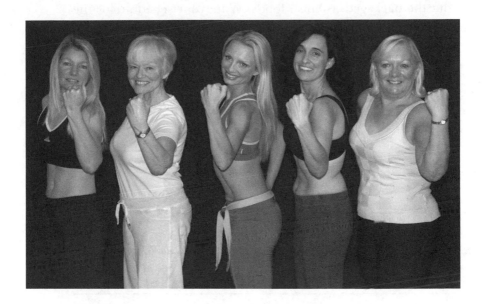

WEEK ONE

TRACEY'S TAKE

Congratulations! You've made the commitment to take care of your body. It's time to stop criticizing the person you see in the mirror and get

TEAM MALLETT'S TAKE

I'm excited about the new plan, but it's going to be very hard to get used to only five servings of grain per day and only four alcohol servings per week. But I'm committed! I've lost weight this week but I need to get serious to get the body I'd like.
—*Desiree Pappenheimer, 28, Boston, Massachusetts*

on the road to feeling hot and sexy. Being prepared is not just for Girl Scouts. It goes for healthy eating, too. Go shopping for your superfoods and toss out the packaged, rubbish foods. Write your schedule for the week because no schedule often means failure. You're on a mission. You're on Team Mallett! I'm excited and you should be, too!

TEAM MALLETT'S TAKE

I am so jazzed about your program! I am energized and motivated to get going.
I still have a long way to go to reach my goal, but I'll get there, thanks to you!
—Valerie Horrey-Wold, 40, South Pasadena, California

WEEK TWO

I'm so surprised at the changes in my body. Not only have I shed 3 1/2 pounds, but my waist looks great. My spare tire is now like one of those little spares you get as opposed to a full-sized tire. I expect it to be gone totally within the next few weeks. I've got quite the two pack and I see the third and fourth of the pack starting to emerge! My clothes all feel great and now I'm eyeing the ones I haven't been able to wear in a while. My husband has commented that my breasts are looking great, which is one of the greatest compliments a 48-year-old woman can get! After fighting gravity all these years, it's nice to know you can do something to make them look rounder and perkier.
—Robin Wood, 48, Fayetteville, North Carolina

TRACEY'S TAKE

You're probably a little sore this week and feeling muscles that you never knew existed. Good job! That's where you want to be. By this time, you should also have a good idea about food portions. At the end of week two, it's time to get on the scale and record your progress. (Remember that in my plan, we weigh ourselves every two weeks.) Don't forget to write down your measurements and how you feel *before* you get on the scale.

_____

_____

_____

_____

TEAM MALLETT'S TAKE

I already look and feel great. I love the encouraging compliments from coworkers! I love the food plan. It's completely changed the way I eat, order, and shop for groceries!
—Alison Fukomoto, 29, Santa Monica, California

WEEK THREE

I realized that I have to do this for myself because I'm really important.
My body is the home for my soul and it needs to be maintained.
It is who I am and that's why I'm not going to give up!
—Sue Giudice, 50, Perth, Australia

TRACEY'S TAKE

Going into the third week, you may be coming down from a natural high of working hard and seeing results. By the end of the week, you may be realizing that this program is a true commitment and a new way of life. You feel a little scared. You don't want to fail. Negative thoughts go through your mind about quitting the program. Am I correct? If not, good for you. Keep up the good work! If I'm onto something, stop those negative thoughts right now! Just think how far you have come. Even just starting the program is a huge leap of faith. Do you realize that most women just sit and procrastinate and never do anything about trying to change their lifestyle? These are the people who pretend to be happy but deep down have little confidence and are searching for peace. As Nike says, "Just do it." You will never look back, I promise!

_____

_____

_____

_____

TEAM MALLETT'S TAKE

I was trying on pants that I bought a few months ago and I can put them on and take them off without unbuttoning them! I'm more excited than I have been in a long time.
—Leanne Scarcella, 29, Rowley, Massachusetts

WEEK FOUR

I fell off the wagon this weekend! I was at a family function where I didn't have much control over my food choices and I am so bloated now. I'm sure it's mostly water retention from all the salt and some alcohol, but I'm now back on track! Exercise is not such a chore anymore. It's just something that's part of my evening routine.
—*Tanya Torforson, 28, Bruderheim, Canada*

TRACEY'S TAKE

I call this week the "hump week" because in the first few weeks you may lose weight quickly, but then your weight loss might slow down or become stagnant. In turn, this can cause discouragement and the first thing you turn to is food. Don't! (Team Mallett had a tough fourth week and some even experienced a few setbacks.) Be aware that this may happen and be ready for it. If or when it does, put your shoes on and go out for a brisk walk or run. No one is perfect. You can do this. Just pretend that any bad moments didn't happen. Also, it's week four, so remember to record your weight and measurements.

_____

_____

_____

_____

_____

TEAM MALLETT'S TAKE

I've been trying to follow your eating plan. Most days are good, but every once in a while I slip. But I am going from not moving at all and eating mindlessly to paying attention to how and what I am eating and trying to move as much as possible.
—*Randy Hsu, 41, Short Hill, New Jersey*

WEEK FIVE

I can't believe there is only one more week to go! Starting out, I figured I'd be on my last legs by the end, but I'm just getting started! I haven't lost any more weight this week, but I felt a big difference in my clothes. Someone commented on my baggy pants and I received several compliments on my little waist. I usually wear my shirts out, but I tucked them in, which I guess made my shape more noticeable. It was just funny to be complimented on the same old outfits I had worn many times before.
—Robin Wood, 48, Fayetteville, North Carolina

TRACEY'S TAKE

You're feeling good right now and starting to see the hard-earned rewards from the program! Yippee! Friends and family members are dishing out the compliments and you feel hot. You should! One of my Team Mallett members, Liz Price, said that by week five, she couldn't stop touching her newfound obliques because she never had them before. "I'm touching my belly like I did when I was pregnant. It feels good," she said.

_____

_____

_____

_____

_____

_____

TEAM MALLETT'S TAKE

I've lost a little over 10 pounds. My clothes are looser and my stomach has gone down a lot.
—Niki Robinson, 33, Fayetteville, Georgia

WEEK SIX

I was thrilled yesterday when I stood on the scale and saw that I had lost 10 pounds!
This is the lightest I've been since I had my first child three years ago! I can't believe
that I am where I am one year after having my second child. The biggest thing your plan
has taught me is to be more aware of what I'm eating. With smaller portions and a
better balance of foods, I feel so much better! All of my "fat clothes" are too big!
I see a good shopping trip of smaller-sized clothes in my near future!
—Jennifer Mahoney, 33, East Norriton, Pennsylvania

TRACEY'S TAKE

The final countdown to a new and healthy you. The plan is now a new way of life. Yes, this is your life! You've read Team Mallett's results throughout the book. They're so inspiring. I can't wait to hear about your healthy transformation, so please e-mail and tell me all about it at tracey@traceymallett.com

_____

_____

_____

_____

_____

TEAM MALLETT'S TAKE

I was in a home improvement store when a college kid who was about
20 years old hit on me, asking me to help him pick out a bed. I smiled but
continued walking to meet my husband and daughter in another part of the store.
The kid followed me and his facial expression when he saw my daughter scream,
"Mommy!" as she ran toward me was worth every sit-up and lunge!
—Leanne Scarcella, 29, Rowley, Massachusetts

The exercises are easy to follow and don't require a huge time commitment. I've lost almost 10 pounds and feel really good about how I look. I've struggled with toning my abs and hips for years and have tried many different diets and exercise plans, but yours is the best. The variety of the workouts allows me to target the areas that need extra work, and I feel stronger and healthier than I have in a long time. I will definitely recommend your book to all my friends. It's excellent!
—Loren Alison, 46, South Pasadena, California

Success Story

· ·

Leanne Scarella, 29, Northeastern, Massachusetts

Lost

10 pounds
8 percent body fat
Two dress sizes
2 inches off her chest
1 inch off her arms
3½ inches off her waist
2 inches off her hips
3½ off inches off her thighs
12 inches total

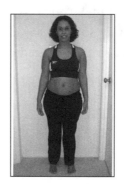
Before

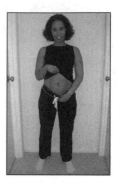
After

Gained

A glass-half-full attitude. *I'm naturally a very pessimistic person, yet now I smile and laugh more rather than moping. Even when I had many more pounds to lose, I had faith that I would make it to the finish line. And that is a*

TEAM MALLETT'S TAKE

Thanks again for everything!! I have learned a lot and am ecstatic to have started a new healthy way of living.
—Christine Alfano, 32, Columbia, Maryland

very positive outlook for me. I truly feel happy from people telling me I have more "life" in me instead of feeling moody from sleep deprivation.

• • • • •

Although Leanne Scarella's "baby" was an 18-month-old toddler, she still hadn't lost all her pregnancy weight. "Before giving birth and becoming a stay-at-home mom, I was a fitness-conscious yoga instructor and dancer. I thought my prior athleticism meant the pregnancy weight would come off instantaneously," says this mother of one. But even eight months post-partum, people were asking Leanne when her baby was due. "I was horrified. But by the time my daughter was a year and a half, I still hadn't lost a pound!" Even worse, she was still wearing maternity clothes. "I was extremely depressed and felt ugly and undeserving of affection from my husband," she says. "I lost all sight of my identity." Leanne needed motivation to help alleviate her "mommy body blues." That came in the form of Tracey's program.

Leanne had never used weights out of fear of bulking up (a common myth). Ironically, it was the strength-training part of Tracey's program that Leanne credits with helping her shed pounds so quickly. In fact, her body changed so much that people were asking for her help. "Women in my building would stop me to ask for my secret, and my mother, who has been overweight her entire life, was so inspired that she started exercising daily and eating better," she says.

Changing her eating also had a big effect on Leanne's ever-slimmer figure. She no longer skipped meals and made them more balanced by eating fewer carbs and more protein. She also learned to satisfy her chocolate cravings with one individually wrapped piece of chocolate— not a whole box or a candy bar. Although she'd always prepared healthy meals, she realized that she never took exact measurements of her ingre-

LEANNE'S STICK-WITH-IT TIP

Have a good support system. It's so helpful to have people around you who are encouraging you. Just one person can keep you from going astray and motivate you when you hit a plateau.

dients. As a result, her portions and calories were way too high. "Taking the time to measure the food while cooking was a huge change," she says.

Just a few weeks into the program, Leanne noticed a difference. "I had so much more energy when I was playing with my daughter. I found myself chasing her around the house instead of just watching her run, and I actually enjoyed being her human jungle gym," she says. These results became her motivation to stick with the program. Her favorite compliment came from her father-in-law. "He told me to be careful or soon I wouldn't have a shadow. I thought that was cute," she says. Today, exercise and healthy eating give Leanne the mood boost she needed. "I'm on my way to meeting my personal goals," she says. "And I feel positive that I can do it."

TRACEY'S TAKE

Leanne has a wonderful spirit. I really felt that she worked so hard not only for herself but also not to let me down. I know Leanne wants to have another baby and was concerned about going into another pregnancy carrying those extra pounds. She did the right thing, and now she has the tools to stay fit during pregnancy. Leanne will have no problems shedding pounds after her next little one is born because she now knows that she can do it!

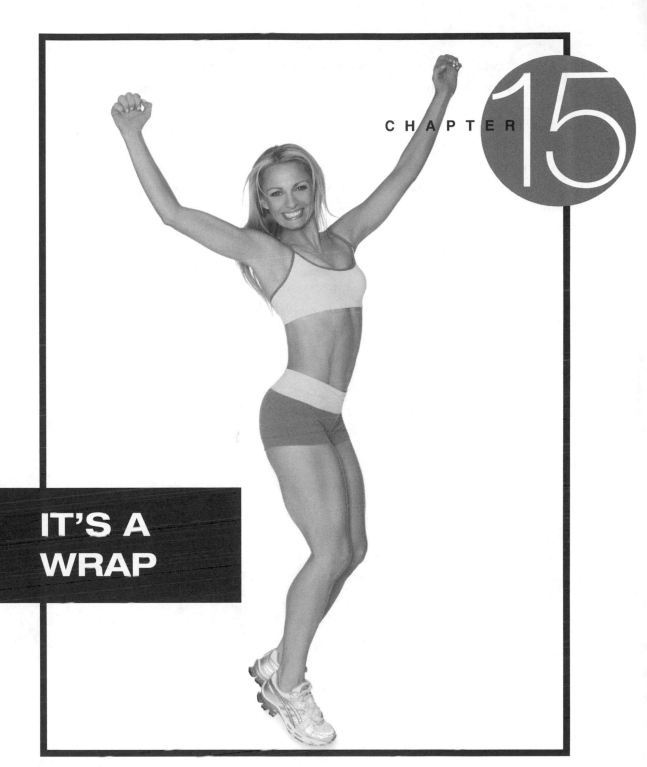

CHAPTER 15

IT'S A WRAP

ONGRATULATIONS! WHETHER YOU ARE JUST STARTING THE *Sexy in 6* program, or are six weeks into it, or are somewhere in between, you should be proud. You have the desire to live a better life and have taken the steps to start that journey. Yes, you're at the end of this book, but you're really at the beginning of a better, healthier, and happier life. The members of Team Mallett all ended their six weeks telling me that they felt as though it was just the beginning, and I agree. In fact, one of them summed it up perfectly. "What one can take away from Team Mallett can be explained with an analogy to flying a plane," says Etta Korenman, age 52. "The *Sexy in 6* plan was the take-off. Now that we are up, we don't stop flying. We keep eating right and exercising (even if some days all we can do is ab work while sitting at a red light in our cars), and we continue the change in our lifestyle. We may hit turbu-

TEN THINGS THAT CAN GIVE YOU A NATURAL HIGH

1. Falling in love

2. Being told you're beautiful

3. The ocean

4. Hearing a song from your college days

5. Laughing at yourself

6. Lying in bed and listening to the rain
(I did this a lot in England)

7. Watching a child sleep

8. Watching the sunset

9. Knowing you did the right thing,
no matter what other people think

10. Waking up and realizing how lucky you are
for another amazing day

lence or have to reroute from time to time, but we don't give up and crash." I couldn't have said it better myself!

The more you practice your good habits, the more they'll become ingrained. They *become* your life, and that is truly the goal. It does not matter whether it takes six days, six weeks, or six months. What does matter is that you're doing it. You'll slip up. I do. We all do. But with the knowledge you now have, you can reach your health and fitness goals.

You're also prepared to feel better in other ways. As I heard over and over from Team Mallett, the benefits of their new lives were far reaching, going beyond looking good in and out of their clothes. I heard their claims of everything from renewed energy and a better attitude to more self-esteem and confidence. I could go on and on (which you know by now because you're used to my chatty style), but I won't.

I will say that when I started writing this book, I was doing it to help other women. But what began as a gift for others truly became a gift for me. I have learned so much about myself writing this book and working with Team Mallett. They say I've inspired them, but they have inspired me a hundred times more. I am so glad to be part of Team Mallett and am thrilled that you are, too. Go team!

I'll leave you with this thought:

"The dream in life is being able to dream."

APPENDIX A:
FOOD LOG, WORKOUT LOG,
AND PROGRESS SHEET

FOOD LOG

	Protein	Dairy	Grains	Fruits	Fats	Veggies (nonstarches)	Water
Breakfast	P P P P	D D	G G	F	FATS	V V V	W W
Snack	P P	D D	G	F F		V V V	W
Lunch	P P P P	D D	G G	F	FATS	V V V	W W
Snack	P P	D D	G	F F		V V V	W
Dinner	P P P P	D D	G G	F	FATS	V V V	W W
Evening snack (optional)	P P	D D	G	F F	FATS	V V V	W
Day's Maximum	7	3	5	4	3	Unlimited	Unlimited

DAY'S TOTAL

Journal Your Treat:

Daily Notes:

REMINDER

Use the food log to monitor your intake. It's easy; just cross off your portion sizes and total them up at the end of the day.

Try not to go over your Day's Maximum!

WORKOUT LOG

	MON	TUES	WED	THUR	FRI	SAT	SUN
A.M.							DAY OFF
LUNCH							
P.M.							
TOTAL QUICK BLASTS							
BONUS CARDIO							
COMMENTS							

Progress Sheet

Fill out the sheet every 2 weeks   Dates/Week # _____ to _____

Beginning Weight: _____   End Weight: _____

How do your clothes feel?

Beginning   *End*

Loose? _____   Tight: _____   Looser? _____   No change: _____

MEASUREMENTS

WAIST

   Beginning: _____   *End:* _____

HIPS

   Beginning: _____   *End:* _____

THIGHS

   Beginning   *End*

   Right: _____   Left: _____   Right: _____   Left: _____

CHEST

   Beginning: _____   *End:* _____

ARMS (in between shoulder & elbow)

   Beginning   *End*

   Right: _____   Left: _____   Right: _____   Left: _____

Energy levels

Beginning: _____   *End:* _____

How do you feel overall?

Beginning: _____   *End:* _____

FISH, SEAFOOD, BEEF, AND POULTRY

Wild Alaskan salmon fillet
Smoked salmon or lox (wild salmon if possible)
Sea scallops
Peeled medium cooked shrimp
Fillet mignon
Chicken tenders
Boneless, skinless chicken breasts
Lean turkey mince meat

PRODUCE

Arugula
Asparagus
Avocado
Baby potatoes
Baby spinach
Banana
Basil
Bean sprouts
Broccoli
Butter lettuce
Carrots
Celery
Chives
Cilantro
Cucumber
Garlic
Ginger
Green bell pepper
Green onions
Jicama
Lemons
Lettuce leaves (Romaine and other types for salads)
Limes
Mango
Mushrooms (white or cremini)
Onions
Oranges
Papaya
Parsley
Pineapple (fresh or frozen)
Red bell pepper

Red onion
Roma tomatoes
Salsa (fresh, often found in the
    produce section)
Snap peas
Strawberries
Sweet potatoes
Tomato (large for stuffing)
Tomatoes, cherry

DAIRY AND SOY

Cheddar cheese, reduced-fat
Cottage cheese, low-fat
Cream cheese, Neufchatel or low-fat
Eggs
Feta cheese, reduced fat
Greek yogurt, low fat
Milk, low-fat
Monterey Jack cheese, reduced fat
Parmesan cheese
Part-skim mozzarella
Sour cream, low-fat
Soy milk, low fat
Soy milk, vanilla
Tofu, firm

GRAINS

Crackers, whole-grain
Croutons, whole-wheat
English muffin, whole-wheat
Hamburger buns, whole-wheat
Pita bread, wheat
Quinoa

Rice, brown
Toast, whole-wheat
Tortillas, whole-grain

CANNED GOODS, CARTONS, BOTTLED GOODS

Black beans
Chicken stock, low-sodium
Green chilies, chopped
Marinara sauce (without sugar or
    low sugar)
Oatmeal (steel cut if possible, but
    rolled oats are fine)
Pinto beans
Pomegranate or apple pomegranate juice
    (may also be fresh)
Refried beans, nonfat vegetarian
Tomatoes, chopped or crushed
Tuna, water-packed
Vegetable stock

FROZEN

Blueberries
Strawberries
Whole-wheat waffles

MISCELLANEOUS ITEMS

Almond butter
Almonds (unsalted)
Basil, dried

Bay leaves

Cayenne pepper

Chile powder

Cocoa powder, unsweetened

Coconut water (available at Whole Foods or other health food stores)

Cumin powder

Dijon mustard

Flaxseeds (available at Whole Foods or other health food stores)

Garlic powder

Ginger, minced crystallized

Ground cinnamon

Honey

Hot sauce (your choice)

Lemon juice

Macadamia nut oil (available at Whole Foods and other stores)

Mayonnaise, reduced-fat

Mirin (Japanese cooking wine)

Olive oil

Oregano, dried

Red pepper flakes

Rice vinegar, seasoned

Sesame oil

Sesame seeds

Shredded coconut, unsweetened

Soy sauce, low-sodium

Vanilla extract

Walnuts

Whey powder (available at Whole Foods or other health food stores)

Worcestershire sauce

ITEMS FOR SNACKS (YOUR CHOICE)

Almonds, pistachios, cashews, or other nuts

Animal crackers

Apples

Cantaloupe

Cheese, low-fat Laughing Cow

Cherries

Chicken noodle soup (less than 350 milligrams of sodium)

Chocolate pudding, low-fat

Cottage cheese, low-fat

Crackers, whole-grain

Edamame (found in the frozen section)

Energy bars

Grapes

Green tea

Honeydew melon

Hummus

Kiwi

Nut butter

Peanut butter (natural is the best option)

Pepitas (pumpkin seeds)

Popcorn (to be air-popped)

Popcorn, air-popped microwavable

Saltine crackers

Soybeans (steamed edamame)

String cheese, low-fat

Sunflower seeds

Tortilla chips, baked

Triscuits, whole wheat

Turkey breast, deli sliced

Wheat Thins, 100-calorie

BALL, FOAM ROLLERS, WEIGHTS, AND MATS

For all your fitness products (balls, foam rollers, weights, and mats), go to

www.optp.com
www.spriproducts.com
www.fitnesswholesale.com

EXERCISE DVDS

Exercise DVDs are a great way of doing your workout without leaving the house. It's like having your own personal trainer in your living room. Team Mallett loved the feeling of working out with me.

This book comes with a sampler DVD of the 6-minute Quick Blast method. The other two DVDs are available for purchase in retail stores and online. Following are Web sites where you can purchase a variety of videos:

www.traceymallett.com
www.amazon.com
www.collage.com
www.razordigitalent.com

I'm looking forward to our workouts!

YUMMY HEALTHY FOODS

As you know, eating healthy is important to me. Here are some of my favorite foods. Check them out. I know you won't be disappointed.

Arnold Natural Flax & Fiber Bread: http://arnold.gwbakeries.com
Dannon Activia Yogurt: www.dannon.com
Drink Hint: www.drinkhint.com
Kookie Karma: www.kookiekarma.com
Lara Bars: www.larabar.com
Vitalicious VitaMuffin: www.vitalicious.com

CLOTHING AND SHOES

In this section are some of my favorite stylish clothes for working out or just for hanging out and looking hot!

www.acicsamerica.com (video)
www.hardtailforever.com (video)
www.lucy.com (inside pictures)
www.rogiani.com (cover)
www.speedo.com (inside pictures)

My favorite running shoes are www.asicsamerica.com. I wore them in the video and in all the pictures in this book.

INFORMATION WEB SITES

Here are some Web sites offering valuable information on health and wellness:

American Academy on Exercise: www.ace.com
Aerobics and Fitness Association of America: www.afaa.com
Ban Trans Fat Information Site: www.bantransfat.com
Centers for Disease Control: www.cdc.gov

Consumer Reports: www.consumerreports.org/healthaccess

Food pyramid: www.mypyramid.gov

National Agricultural Library (SDA Nutrient Database): www.nal.usda.gov

WebMD: www.webmd.com

DOWNLOADABLE WORKOUTS

Go to www.iamplify.com to download my workouts. Save 30 percent when you use the promotion code tracey1.

VIDEO ON DEMAND

Check your local cable listing for *Exercise TV,* where you can find hundreds of workouts to choose from, including mine.

MY CONTRIBUTOR FRIENDS

Please check out these amazing people who generously contributed to my book.

Carilyn Vaile

Carilyn Vaile (www.carilynvaile.com) is a fashion designer and the author of *I Am Diva! Every Woman's Guide to Outrageous Living* (Warner Books). She not only brings peace to the busy woman's daily outfit drama, but also designs pieces that work for them in a variety of flattering and fashion-forward ways. And her creative commando approach to wardrobe reinvention has made her a favorite fashion spokesperson on television and in print, nationwide.

Dr. Ava Cadell

Love guru, media therapist, author and world-class speaker, Dr. Ava Cadell (www.avacadell.com) is an accomplished author of seven books. Dr. Ava has a doctorate in human behavior from Newport University,

California, and a doctorate of education in human sexuality from the Institute for Advanced Study of Human Sexuality in San Francisco. Through her private practice in Los Angeles, she counsels people on personal issues, including anger management, lack of communication, fear of intimacy, and lack of desire.

Chantal Donnelly, MPT, CMT

A faculty member for the Physical Therapy Department at Mount St. Mary's College in Los Angeles, Chantal Donnelly (www.bodyinsight101.com) is currently working on some exciting Pilates research. She is also the creator and owner of Body Insight, a rehabilitation company dedicated to producing fun, innovative exercise videos for people with specific pain problems. Her newest video is "Knees 101."

Howard Kaufman, MD, MBA

Howard Kaufman (www.surgery.usc.edu) is Associate Professor of Surgery and Obstetrics and Gynecology, and Chief, Division of Colorectal and Pelvic Floor Surgery at Keck School of Medicine, University of Southern California; Director, USC Pelvic Floor Disorders Program; and Chief, General Surgery at USC University Hospital.

Jonny Bowden, Ph.D., C.N.S.

Jonny Bowden (www.jonnybowden.com) is the author of the best-selling *Living the Low Carb Life: Choosing the diet that's right for you from Atkins to Zone* (Sterling Books, 2004). His new book is *The 150 Best Foods on Earth* (Fair Winds Press).

Lisa Delaney

Lisa Delaney (www.formerfatgirl.com), author of *Secrets of a Former Fat Girl: How to Drop Two, Four (or More!) Dress Sizes—and Find Yourself Along the Way,* is an award-winning magazine writer and editor and is currently special projects director at *Health* magazine.

I have to be honest. When I first accepted the offer to write this book, I had no idea how many people and how many sleepless nights it would take to put a book together. There's no way I could take "all the" credit for this book. So many amazing people were involved with this project and I really couldn't have done it without them. (I feel like I'm writing my Oscar acceptance speech!)

So here goes. Linda Konner, my literary agent who made all of this happen. She found me a great partner in Da Capo Press, which I'm thrilled to be working with.

Michele Bender, my partner in crime, who truly is a master with words. Thank you from the bottom of my heart, we truly make a good team. This book would not be the same without you!

Christy Hedges, Wendy Crump, and Sharon Richter, for their valuable nutritional suggestions. You're the best!

My husband, Chris, for lots of extra babysitting. I know he's as happy as I am now that the book is finished. Thank you and I love you.

Matthew Lore, Katie McHugh, and everyone at Da Capo Press and Christine Marra of Marrathon Production Services for their constant support and belief in this project from day one. Dorit Theis, whose beautiful photography made this book complete.

My dearest friends Cal Pozo, James Flint, Stacey Hanson, Chantal Donnelly, and Kimberly Spencer for their ongoing pillars of support and guidance on this project. I love you guys!

Team Mallett, my true heartbeat and inspiration for this book. Thank you for opening up to me and facing your fears. Your stories are so inspirational and motivational. Thank you, thank you, and thank you!

I also want to thank ASICS and Speedo, generous sponsors of the book and video.

Last but not least, my Mom and Dad, for always telling me from when I was a young child, "You can do it." Thank you for believing in me even when I doubted myself.

Kisses to my kids, Amber and Ty, for making me realize how lucky I am to be their Mommy.

Tracey's Companion Super Fat Blasting DVDs

Let Tracey motivate you to success right from your living room! These workouts are taken directly from *Sexy in 6*—if you love this program, you won't want to miss out on these new 6 Minute Quick*Blast* Method DVDs.

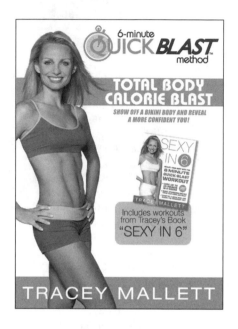 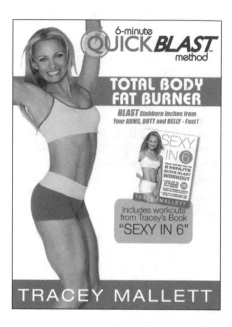

- 6 Minute Quick*Blasts,* so you can work out on YOUR terms when YOU have time
- Total Body Sculpting AND Calorie Fat Blasting workouts
- A proven program by the women who have lost pounds, inches and dress sizes who are quoted in this book.
- Choose your own custom workout for your body type and put it to action with these DVDs today!

To purchase, visit www.traceymallett.com or www.amazon.com.

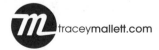